PLANNED MARKETS AND
PUBLIC COMPETITION

STATE OF HEALTH SERIES

Edited by Chris Ham, Fellow in Health Policy and Management, King's Fund College

Current and forthcoming titles

Hospitals in Transition
Tim Packwood, Justin Keen and Martin Buxton

Planned Markets and Public Competition
Richard B. Saltman and Casten von Otter

Accountability in the NHS
Diane Longley

Financing Health Care in the 1990s
John Appleby

PLANNED MARKETS AND PUBLIC COMPETITION

Strategic Reform in Northern European Health Systems

Richard B. Saltman and Casten von Otter

Open University Press
Buckingham · Philadelphia

Open University Press
Celtic Court
22 Ballmoor
Buckingham
MK18 1XW

and

1900 Frost Road, Suite 101
Bristol, PA 19007, USA

First Published 1992

A catalogue record of this book is
available from the British Library

Library of Congress Cataloging-in-Publication Data

Saltman, Richard B.
    Planned markets and public competition: strategic reform in northern
European health systems/by Richard Saltman and Casten von Otter.
        p.   cm. – (The State of health series)
    ISBN 0–335–09728–6 (pbk.)   ISBN 0–335–09729–4 (cased)
    1. Medical economics – Europe, Northern.   2. Medical care –
Europe, Northern – Marketing.   3. Health planning – Europe,
Northern.
    I. Otter, Casten von, 1941–   .   II. Title.   III. Series.
    (DNLM: 1. Delivery of Health Care – economics – Europe.
2. Economic Competition – organization & administration – Europe.
3. Economic Competition – trends – Europe.   4. Marketing of Health
    Services.   W74 S178p]
    RA410.9.E853S26   1992
    362.1′094 – dc20
    DNLM/DLC
    for Library of Congress   91–46379
                                                                        CIP

Typeset by Type Study, Scarborough
Printed in Great Britain by St Edmundsbury Press,
Bury St Edmunds, Suffolk

HMT
dw
S

91   10193

CONTENTS

SERIES EDITOR'S INTRODUCTION

Health services in many developed countries have come under critical scrutiny in recent years. In part this is because of increasing expenditure, much of it funded from public sources, and the pressure this has put on governments seeking to control public spending. Also important has been the perception that resources allocated to health services are not always deployed in an optimal fashion. Thus at a time when the scope for increasing expenditure is extremely limited, there is a need to search for ways of using existing budgets more efficiently. A further concern has been the desire to ensure access to health care of various groups on an equitable basis. In some countries this has been linked to a wish to enhance patient choice and to make service providers more responsive to patients as 'consumers'.

Underlying these specific concerns are a number of more fundamental developments which have a significant bearing on the performance of health services. Three are worth highlighting. First, there are demographic changes, including the ageing population and the decline in the proportion of the population of working age. These changes will both increase the demand for health care and at the same time limit the ability of health services to respond to this demand.

Second, advances in medical science will also give rise to new demands within the health services. These advances cover a range of possibilities, including innovations in surgery, drug therapy, screening and diagnosis. The pace of innovation is likely to quicken as the end of the century approaches, with significant implications for the funding and provision of services.

Third, public expectations of health services are rising as those who use services demand higher standards of care. In part, this is stimulated by developments within the health service, including the availability of new technology. More fundamentally, it stems from the emergence of a more educated and informed population, in which people are accustomed to being treated as consumers rather than patients.

Against this background, policymakers in a number of countries are reviewing the future of health services. Those countries which have traditionally relied on a market in health care are making greater use of regulation and planning. Equally, those countries which have traditionally relied on regulation and planning are moving towards a more competitive approach. In no country is there complete satisfaction with existing methods of financing and delivery, and everywhere there is a search for new policy instruments.

The aim of this series is to contribute to debate about the future of health services through an analysis of major issues in health policy. These issues have been chosen because they are both of current interest and of enduring importance. The series is intended to be accessible to students and informed lay readers as well as to specialists working in this field. The aim is to go beyond a textbook approach to health policy analysis and to encourage authors to move debate about their issue forward. In this sense, each book presents a summary of current research and thinking, and an exploration of future policy directions.

Dr Chris Ham
Fellow in Health Policy and Management
King's Fund College

PREFACE

The health policy debate in Northern Europe is increasingly focused on the question of the introduction of competition into publicly operated delivery systems. The potential advantages and disadvantages of such a shift have come to dominate discussion among not only academics but also politicians, administrators and now physicians and patients as well. There appears to be little danger in predicting that this issue will strongly influence the development of Northern European health policy through much of the 1990s.

Despite consensus on the importance of the topic, there is little apparent agreement on the precise meaning of the concept of competition itself. Different health sector actors have chosen to define the term in fundamentally different ways, seeking to emphasize those particular aspects of market-based systems that appear most likely to strengthen their particular group's own negotiating position. As a consequence, the current debate has occasionally served more to obfuscate rather than illuminate key underlying issues involved in such a structural reorganization.

The introduction of competition into heretofore publicly operated health systems continues to be a highly controversial strategy. Various health sector actors, having defined the concept differently, also tend to read their own fears and preferences into the particular version that they perceive on the political horizon. Those opposed to competitive approaches cite a long and important list of concerns, revolving in substantial measure around questions of equity and access on the one hand, and the maintenance of preventive, primary and public health programmes, on the other. Similarly, proponents of competitive models – and those who view competitive arrangements more as inevitable than ideal – anticipate more positive but equally particular outcomes from this policy shift. While a number of physicians and other health professionals tend to view competitive mechanisms as a way to increase both professional autonomy and salaries, many managers view competition as a framework to push medical personnel to adopt more efficient working patterns. While a substantial number of patients anticipate that competition will increase their range of provider and treatment alternatives, health sector managers often see competitive mechanisms as instruments to steer patients toward less expensive providers. Finally, and most potentially fraught, while individual entrepreneurs typically see competition as the road to personal financial success, most politicians view competition as an arrangement to reduce overall health care expenditures.

While competition can perhaps be all things to all people in theory, it clearly cannot remain so if it is to be put into practice. In most Northern European health systems, the key policy questions surrounding the implementation of a competition-based approach have yet to be decided. Among other essential issues (Saltman *et al.*, 1991), one could raise the following. In what subsectors of the delivery system will competitive mechanisms be introduced? Which market incentives will be incorporated: will competition be based on price, on quality or on market share? Which actors will be subject to these incentives? Who will take decisions about capital investment? How will overall standards and quality be maintained? How will producer domination of the regulatory process (often termed 'regulatory capture') and other perverse outcomes be forestalled?

In this book, we develop a conceptual framework that can help interested citizens as well as scholars and policy-makers to place these narrowly economic problems of 'market design' into the broader social and political context that they inevitably reflect. We argue that publicly operated health systems are poised at the edge of a new policy paradigm, a new conceptual framework for delivering health services, which we term 'planned markets'. This planned market paradigm combines elements of both planning and market approaches to health system organization, but in a complementary rather than confrontational configuration. At present, several different types of planned market models are under development, either in service delivery experiments (in Sweden) or in new legislation to restructure existing service arrangements (UK and

Finland). How this process of paradigm creation develops – and the particular combination of public and private forms of health care responsibility that it adopts – will strongly influence the future of publicly operated health systems not only in Northern but most probably in Southern and Eastern Europe as well.

We present our analysis in two closely related segments. In Part I, we review the successes and travails of both publicly operated health systems and of the welfare state more generally over the past several decades. Taking a critical yet sympathetic stance, we assess past and existing organizational processes in both health care and human services sectors in terms of the structural limitations that we believe preclude achievement of stated policy objectives. Subsequently, we explore the hybrid territory between politics and markets that we label 'planned markets'. After setting out the political and normative dimensions that contextualize market decisions *sui generis*, we explore the range of current health sector experimentation with hybrid public–private approaches in publicly operated health systems in the UK, Sweden and Finland. We then review the types of planned markets that currently exist within these three countries, analysing their current stage of direction and development.

In Part II, we present our argument in favour of one specific form of planned market, which we term 'public competition'. We begin with a theoretical justification of our reliance upon patient choice as the driving force within our hybrid model, consistent with what we call 'civil democracy' in public sector human services. We subsequently develop our specific organizational proposal, both as a theory of public markets composed of 'public firms' and in practical administrative terms as an integrated system of health service providers. The volume concludes with an overview of the role which a public competition model, properly configured, might play in the search for a new health sector paradigm over the next decade.

This monograph evolved from a series of individual projects and papers. Two articles appeared in *Health Policy*: 'Re-vitalizing public health systems: a proposal for public competition in Sweden' was published in 1987 (volume 7, no. 1) and 'Public competition vs. mixed markets: an analytic comparison' in 1989 (volume 11, no. 1). We also wish to thank the European Healthcare Management Association, which, in awarding the first Jan Blanpain Prize to our 1987 *Health Policy* article, stimulated us to develop our ideas further. A third article, 'Voice, choice, and the question of civil democracy in the Swedish welfare state', appeared in *Economic and Industrial Democracy* in 1989 (volume 10, no. 2), and a fourth, 'Implementing public competition in Swedish county councils: a case study', was published in the *International Journal of Health Planning and Management* in 1990 (volume 5, no. 2). A fifth article, 'Toward a Swedish health policy in the 1990s: planned markets and public firms', appeared in *Social Science and Medicine* in 1991 (volume 32, no. 4). A Swedish presentation of our ideas, 'Vitalisering av den offentliga sjukvården – Ett förslag till institutionell konkurrens', was published by *Läkartidningen* in 1988 (volume 85). Earlier versions of these articles were presented at annual conferences of the European Healthcare Management Association (1987, 1988, 1989), at the European Health Policy Forum in Brussels (1987) and at an OECD/IULA Workshop in Amsterdam (1988).

Funding for the research and writing of this volume came from a variety of sources. The major burden was defrayed by a research fellowship (to R.B.S.) from the German Marshall Fund of the United States, and from the Public Sector Research Program of the LOM Project (for C.v.O.) sponsored by the Swedish Work Environment Fund. Additional support was provided by two Fulbright Fellowships from the Finland–United States Educational Foundation (to R.B.S.) and by the Health Services Research Unit of the National Public Health Institute of Finland, the Department of Public Health at the University of Helsinki, the Department of Nursing and Health Administration at the University of Kuopio, the Swedish Center for Working Life, the Nordic School of Public Health and the University of Massachusetts at Amherst.

The thinking in this volume reflects discussions with friends and colleagues over the past five years. We particularly wish to thank Andrew Martin of MIT and Harvard. Additional thanks are due to Chris Ham, who read the manuscript in penultimate form and suggested important improvements. S. Åke Lindgren, Gunnar Wennström, Ilkka Vohlonen, Kimmo Leppo, Seppo Aro, Johan Calltorp, Lennart Köhler, Douglas Skalin, Kurt-Lennart Spetz, Per-Olof Brogren, Vibeke Reimer, Per-Gunnar Svensson, Jan Blanpain, Ray Robinson, Herbert Zöllner and Karin Tengvald were important sources of intellectual support over the life of the project. We also like to acknowledge the inspiration provided by Professor Borgonovi's group at Bocconi University in Milan, as well as by numerous Spanish colleagues. We are indebted to Lena

Joelsson, Peter Richman, Kirsten Söderholm and Bengt Åkermalm for research support, and to Yesi Sait, Birgit Larsson and Anna Fundin for excellent secretarial assistance. Finally, we would like to thank our families – Denise, Julian and Annika; and Karin, Salomon, Clara and Cecilia. While none of the above is accountable for the use to which we put their efforts, we are very grateful to them all.

PART I

THE SEARCH FOR A POLICY PARADIGM

1

THE STRATEGIC CROSSROADS

The 1980s was a difficult decade for publicly operated health systems in Northern Europe. Many traditional assumptions about their mission and methods were undermined by a seemingly endless succession of organizational and structural dilemmas. Constructed upon technical or rational planning models that emphasized uniform services and centralized command-and-control decision-making, publicly operated systems faced insistent pressures to differentiate services to different patient groups and to decentralize administrative decision-making to local institutions. Founded upon principles of social justice and demographic entitlement, public health systems were subjected to intense scrutiny based upon neo-classical economic criteria and market-oriented values. Financially dependent upon severely constrained public sector budgets, these systems were expected to provide an expanding volume of high quality curative, custodial and preventive services. Politically dependent upon widespread support to maintain their universal orientation, publicly operated systems experienced a growing lack of popular understanding about their central purposes and objectives.

This increasingly unstable situation was all the more striking given the standards and accomplishments of the health care systems it affects. By most comparative measures, Northern Europe contains some of the most successful health care systems in the developed world. Finland, Sweden, Norway, Denmark and the United Kingdom rank high in terms of access, quality and comprehensiveness of acute clinical and also preventive and custodial services. At the same time, these health systems have controlled their aggregate expenditure levels, spending roughly consistent (in the case of Sweden, falling) proportions of their gross domestic product throughout the 1980s (Schieber and Poullier, 1991). Indeed, this combination of high health status and stable expenditures is often cited by defenders of existing publicly operated systems as clear evidence of their overall effectiveness.

The causal forces behind the present organizational disarray go well beyond short-term financial and political factors. The degree of external pressure for reform does not, for example, appear to reflect a system's basic level of financial resources. Publicly operated systems are experiencing similar difficulties despite levels of aggregate health expenditure which ranged in 1989 from 5.8 per cent of GDP in the United Kingdom to 7.1 per cent in Finland and 8.8 per cent in Sweden (Schieber and Poullier, 1991). Nor are the present problems readily explained by the political beliefs or strength of the sitting national government. At the time of writing, the United Kingdom is ruled by a strong conservative party, Finland by a strong left–right coalition (social democrats and conservatives), and Sweden by a weak left minority government (social democrats working variously with centre, liberal and communist parties).

The unconvincing character of short-term financial and political explanations points to the central importance of more deep-seated structural problems. Viewed historically, publicly operated health systems have been part of the accepted political landscape in Northern Europe since the end of the Second World War. In the initial decades following the war's conclusion, these systems grew at a rapid pace, pursuing as their central goal the attainment of universal access to comprehensive care. The driving force in publicly operated health systems, as in the emerging welfare states of which they were an important component, was normative in character, seeking to extend coverage and services on grounds of social justice and moral obligation. Although this process was often uneven, with health sector proponents obligated to justify each incremental addition on its own merits, the broad thrust of policy development in most countries was consistently normative and expansionary (Flora, 1986–7; Korpi, 1989). While the emphasis upon building new curative facilities, particularly hospitals, would later be criticized by advocates of primary and preventive care, the sheer scope of the expansion gave witness to the period's universal aspirations.

The dominant health policy paradigm during this post-war

expansion was a relatively rigid command-and-control planning model. Decision-making responsibility was formally vested in elected officials at national (the UK), national and regional (Sweden, Denmark, Norway) or national and municipal (Finland) levels, while day-to-day operating authority was delegated by these politicians to a corps of career administrators and planners. This top-down planning model was conceptualized as a publicly accountable arrangement that could ensure provision of a necessary social good in a universal and hence cost-effective fashion. As aggregate health statistics over the past three decades clearly demonstrate, these publicly planned systems have been broadly successful in achieving this objective. Indeed, in the 1980s, to the extent that Northern European countries have required fewer financial resources (with the exception of Sweden, substantially fewer resources) than countries with mixed public/private or pluralist health systems (such as Germany, France, the Netherlands or the United States) despite (with the exception of the UK) an equivalent growth in per capita income and national wealth, the top-down planning model has proved itself to be still an effective instrument for aggregate health system development.

Despite this continued good performance at an overall system level, severe and seemingly intractable problems with centralized planning models emerged during the 1970s and 1980s at the institutional and individual patient level. Health planning models typically require a stable environment in order to perform well: a stable knowledge base regarding the services to be provided; a stable organizational and equipment base from which to deliver those services; a stable personnel base to staff those facilities; and stable expectations from patients as to the services they will receive. It is stability that allows long-term planning to allocate resources and personnel in accordance with a rational or technical approach to service delivery. Unfortunately, precisely this core assumption of stability fell by the wayside during the 1970s and 1980s. Diagnostic and therapeutic procedures changed rapidly because of advances in basic medical science; new forms of expensive capital equipment progressed from experimental to routine usage by hospital specialists; rapid growth in the number of elderly citizens required expanded rehabilitative, custodial and home care services; increased mobility in the workforce generally (and rising wages in the private sector in particular) generated labour unrest among health sector workers; and an increasingly affluent citizenry became less willing to accept services delivered on the provider's rather than the patient's terms.

Further, the process of administration during the prior period of stability had ossified into a state of formalized rigidity. The consequences of organizational petrification included: administrative regulations for fixed institutional budgets and personnel salaries with strong disincentives for higher productivity; a retrospective reimbursement process for out-of-district services which often took two years to complete, creating additional disincentives for efficient utilization of resources;[1] and a counterproductive combination of strong provider pressures – often exercised through labour unions – and minimal patient influence, which served to reinforce a process of 'regulatory capture' in which provider interests dominated the planning agenda (Long, 1949).

The inability of traditional planning models to deal effectively with the emerging situation was underscored further by a major shift in the conceptual lens through which Western capitalist states came to view public activity generally. By the late 1970s and early 1980s, the logic of neo-classical economics had begun to replace that of classical democratic politics as the core theoretical basis upon which to evaluate all types of social activity. Markets were increasingly seen to embody the virtues that politics, and with it public sector organization, appeared to lack. Reflecting this broad societal trend, the language of health policy formulation and evaluation also changed. Although neo-classical models were initially developed for use within pluralist, insurance-based health systems like that found in the United States (Greenberg, 1978; Enthoven, 1980), the new policy paradigm soon challenged existing organizational assumptions within publicly operated health systems as well. In this changed conceptual environment, planning models could no longer be justified solely on their ability to provide universal services and to enhance social justice. In their stead, economists' assumptions about productivity rapidly became the pre-eminent criteria for judging the appropriateness of clinical and preventive services.

Like other shifts in a dominant conceptual paradigm (Kuhn, 1962), this change in the underlying assumptions about health policy was precipitated by a series of trigger events. In this instance, those events were economic: the oil shock of 1973, followed by nearly a decade of so-called 'stagflation' (stagnant economic growth combined with inflation). This 'end to growth', and with it the end to associated increases in tax revenues, forced central governments across Northern Europe to rein in public sector spending sharply. As a consequence, in publicly operated as well as in pluralist health care systems in Europe, health officials and administrators felt increasingly constrained to define organizational objectives in terms of cost-effectiveness categories such as service productivity and delivery efficiency.

The emergence of neo-classical economics as the core frame of policy reference has had certain benefits for publicly operated health systems. Discussions about the internal efficiency of provider organizations, for example, or the responsiveness of service provision to patient desires, have become more focused as a result of economically informed analysis. Similarly, in applied areas like personnel management and information systems, the neo-classical paradigm has raised valuable (if often controversial) questions about system design and implementation.

Neo-classical economics has been rather less useful in highlighting specific mechanisms developed in the USA that can be used within Northern Europe's differently configured health care systems. Concepts like diagnostic related groups (DRGs) and health maintenance organizations (HMOs) were designed to reduce unnecessary expenditures and enhance budget predictability within an insurance-based, fee-for-service delivery system (Håkansson *et al.* 1988). As a result, many of these mechanisms are largely inappropriate within the context of the tax-based, globally budgeted health systems of Northern Europe. In this context, it should be noted that in the United States itself the implementation of a reform strategy based upon neo-classical economics – in which these mechanisms play a key role – has generated sufficient economic as well as clinical havoc (Himmelstein *et al.*, 1989; Schieber and Poullier, 1989) that some originators of competition-based models in the United States now recognize that pure neo-classical principles cannot provide suitable models for health sector reconstruction in industrialized societies (Enthoven, 1989).

The most serious difficulty with attempts to apply the neo-classical paradigm within Northern Europe is the contradiction between the paradigm's central operating premise and the normative objectives that continue to animate publicly operated health systems. The neo-classical paradigm's assumptions about rational decision-making, and particularly its model of a 'rational economic person' who has, among other resources, perfect information and complete decision-making freedom (unencumbered by historical, cultural, social or organizational references), runs directly contrary to both the mission and the actual circumstances of the largest patient base within publicly operated health systems (Etzioni, 1988). As some market-oriented theorists have noted (Enthoven, 1986), the elderly, the young, the chronically ill and the poor have neither the economic resources nor, often, the requisite interest or skills to apply neo-classical notions of rational self-interest to their own benefit. Thus those most in the need of services are the very population that will be worst served by the unfettered market-driven model to which the neo-classical paradigm points (Granqvist, 1987). Additional dilemmas with market conceptions of the health sector include reliance on clinically counterproductive self-diagnosis through mechanisms like cost-sharing and deductible payments (Young and Saltman, 1985), an emphasis upon curative individual-based at the expense of preventive population-based services, and the substitution of legal contract for social contract definitions of medical responsibilities. The inappropriateness of the pure neo-classical paradigm for use within the health sector generally has been acknowledged by several respected health economists. Robert Evans, for example, has written scathingly of 'those who still find the economic theory of the perfectly competitive marketplace a plausible way of thinking about medical care', dismissing such economists as caught up in a 'religion' in which the 'liturgy is . . . expressed in the peculiar jargon of economic analysis' (Evans, 1986).

The liabilities that accompany neo-classical economic logic strongly suggest that it is unable to provide an appropriate replacement paradigm upon which to order health policy decision-making within publicly operated systems. Much like the prior planning paradigm of which it is so critical, the neo-classical economic paradigm fails to accommodate the unique mix of normative, clinical and financial concerns that an appropriately configured health system must address. Given this conceptual failure, its not surprising that health sector officials in most Northern European countries (with the partial exception of the United Kingdom) are unwilling to rely upon the neo-classical approach as a replacement for the acknowledged limitations of the existing command-and-control planning paradigm.

This inability to adopt a strictly market-based solution has left health sector officials in something of a conceptual quandary. Unable to continue with a planning-based logic that has become anachronistic, they none the less recognize the narrowness and inadequacy of the only major policy paradigm put forward as a potential replacement. Faced with impossible alternatives, publicly operated systems have had great difficulty in deciding to choose at all. The result, as the 1980s came to a close, was a palpable loss of organizational and managerial direction. Confronted with powerful pressures from their external environments, no longer able to presume the stable structural foundation required by an allocative planning-based paradigm, yet unwilling to consign themselves to a socially as well as organizationally inappropriate neo-classical economic paradigm, publicly operated systems in Northern Europe have slipped their conceptual moorings without a clear theoretical basis upon which to construct their future. Neither past planning nor present neo-classical economic paradigms will suffice, yet the outline of a new dominant policy paradigm has yet to become visible.

This process of paradigm change is neither voluntary nor driven by particular ideological conditions. Rather, a series of deeply rooted political, social and economic forces have combined to generate essentially similar needs for broad welfare state change regardless of short-run national health-sector preferences.

First, politically, the traditional working class is shrinking and labour unions are losing their ability to form effective political coalitions (Korpi, 1989). As a consequence, publicly provided human services – in particular health services – will survive only if they can be reconfigured to be broadly acceptable to the middle class. Second, socially, younger groups within the middle class, as the affluent 'children of the welfare state', will no longer accept centrally planned human services on a uniform industrial model. Whether one interprets these new expectations positively (in Maslow's framework of new needs (Maslow, 1943)) or more critically (as new-age selfishness), publicly operated health systems have little choice but to restructure themselves to meet these new demands. Third, economically, and perhaps most importantly in historical terms, Western economies are becoming predominantly service rather than manufacturing based. As a result, continued economic prosperity will depend on achieving regular productivity increases in the service sector, and particularly in its largest component, public sector human services. To achieve such increases, publicly operated health services clearly require new modes of organization and management.

The present period of organizational and structural uncertainty is likely to be a prelude to the emergence of a new more appropriate policy paradigm for publicly operated health systems. To borrow a Hegelian framework, the 'thesis' of health planning and the 'antithesis' of neo-classical economics may yet trigger a 'synthesis' which can integrate both prior health system paradigms into a comprehensive and cohesive theoretical construct. This synthesis could provide a firm conceptual basis for the process of 'strategic reform' which publicly operated health systems now require – 'strategic' in that it sets into motion dynamic processes which force a thoroughgoing organizational reconstruction rather than a 'reform-ist reform' which only patches up flaws in existing institutional arrangements (Gorz, 1964). An alternative way to conceptualize strategic reform is that it would generate a process of 'creative restruction' within publicly operated health services similar to but without the social consequences associated with Schumpeter's (1934) notion of 'creative destruction'.

An effective process of strategic reform ought to trigger a broad set of changes in the core characteristics of service delivery institutions. Improved internal efficiency within provider insti-tutions would be integrally connected, indeed driven by, concerns for increased external effectiveness. Budgetary linkages among hospital, primary care and social services would encourage greater continuity of care in the least expensive appropriate facility. Health providers would find it essential to temper tendencies towards professional dominance with individual patients' increased influ-ence, perhaps control, over the treatment process and site.

A new policy paradigm which could attain, or at least asymp-totically approach, these goals could secure the future of publicly operated health systems well into the twenty-first century. It would harness the analytic power of neo-classical economics in the service of, rather than in confrontation with, the traditional normative values that inform publicly operated health systems. Health econ-omics as a particular form of technical expertise could then find its appropriate place, to use Gulick's (1937) classic phrase, 'on tap not on top'.

The process of paradigm shift, however, is complicated and time-consuming. After sufficient evidence has accumulated to document the inadequacies of the current theory, a drawn-out political phase occurs in which alternative theories pursue the consensus necessary to confirm the emergence of a new paradigm (Kuhn, 1962). In publicly operated health systems in Northern Europe, the search for the new paradigm has only just begun, so the precise outlines of the new health policy paradigm are unknown. In the next chapter, we detail the specific problems that the prior command-and-control paradigm can no longer resolve, and then stitch different health systems' fragmentary and/or partial responses together into a general picture of what the new replacement paradigm might eventually look like.

NOTE

1 This was a particular problem in the United Kingdom, where the RAWP (Resource Allocation Working Party) formula was poorly suited to out-of-district payments (Brazier, 1987; Bevan, 1988).

2

THE EMERGENCE OF PLANNED MARKETS

The structural dilemmas of the post-industrial welfare state are painfully visible within publicly operated health systems in Northern Europe. On the one hand, demands for new resources continue to grow unabated. Acute care hospitals require major new investments if they are to stay current with rapidly improving technologies and to provide a high standard of service to the increasing proportion of elderly citizens. Primary and preventive care initiatives – typically initiated during the 1970s and 1980s as a way to reduce aggregate long-term health expenditures – also require infusions of fresh funds if they are to achieve their objectives. Yet national governments remain financially constrained by the economic legacies of the 1970s, in particular by the consequences of having expanded public sector spending during a period of overall economic stagnation. A key objective of macroeconomic policy during the last half of the 1980s, in Social Democratic Sweden as in Tory England, has been to reduce real human services spending overall, so as to increase the available resources for private sector expansion. This pattern, begun during the expansionary years of the 1980s, seems likely to intensify in the recessionary economy of the early 1990s.

The inevitable clash between service-generated demands for new resources and a macroeconomic imperative to reduce spending has generated broad pressure on health institutions to rethink their organizational and delivery patterns. Confronted by the necessity of across-the-board fiscal restraint, Northern European governments have refused to commit large new resources to what they perceive as expensive and inefficient health care systems. Instead, governments have become insistent that their health systems find ways to become more productive with existing resources and personnel. In making these demands, government officials have often cited the results from studies of long-term productivity development in health care, which typically show falling rates over the 1970s and 1980s as treatment patterns for acute health services became more intensive (Finansdepartmentet, 1985; Vohlonen and Pekurinen, 1990).

In addition to financial pressures, there have been increasing calls for publicly operated health systems to improve their responsiveness to patient concerns. Patients have become increasingly vocal in their opposition to continued rationing by queue of certain elective surgical procedures, particularly those performed on elderly patients. Similarly, patients have become less tolerant of health system practices that steer treatment patterns in directions that reflect the health provider's, rather than the individual patient's, treatment preferences. Finally, patients are less willing to accept passively the costs imposed upon them by a variety of logistical factors, such as long waiting-room times, inconvenient appointment hours (i.e. during regular working time), complicated regulations regarding delivery sites, poorly coordinated services and so forth. These and other related patient concerns have led several recent studies to comment upon the perceived powerlessness of the patient within the British and Swedish health care systems (Ham, 1988; Petersson *et al.*, 1989).

A third source of pressure comes from health system employees and employee unions (Heidenheimer and Johansen, 1985). Although specific issues vary in different countries, health employees typically want not just increased salaries but also more interactive participation in managerial decision-making, reductions in the length of the working week and increased resources for health service development and growth. In Sweden, for example, a codetermination process termed MBL (after the law which established it) was introduced to the national labour market in 1977, requiring health administrators to consult affected employees before initiating changes in work routines (von Otter, 1983). In Finland, health sector unions succeeded in 1988 in reducing the standard working week to 37.5 hours, a change that created the need for an estimated 3000 new hospital staff in an otherwise tightly rationed delivery structure (Saltman, 1988a). In 1988 and 1989 in the UK, nursing and physician associations vociferously insisted that the government allocate additional resources and increase available service within the National Health Service (Ham *et al.*, 1990). In all three countries, physicians and particularly nurses have initiated labour actions – including slow-downs, walk-outs and strikes – in support of similar demands.

Despite these multiple pressures, Northern European health policy-makers have often been unable to respond adequately because of the limitations of the traditional command-and-control planning mechanisms with which they have had to work. In the United Kingdom, the centrally administered RAWP (Resource Allocation Working Party) formula for distributing the National Health Service's budget has been criticized as a cumbersome mechanism that does not adequately facilitate either patient flows or treatment patterns (Brazier, 1987; Bevan, 1988). In Finland, the highly detailed national health planning process, which played a central role in developing a strong primary health care sector (Pekurinen *et al.*, 1987), also limited municipal efforts to develop innovative patient management techniques. In Sweden, administrative boundaries between clinical care, social care, social insurance and pharmaceutical reimbursement severely restricted the ability of county councils to manage overall health-related expenditures. In all three countries, a constellation of additional rigidities, including nationally negotiated labour contracts, input-oriented budgets and Weberian bureaucratic regulations as well as arbitrary intervention by political officials (Weber, 1947), served further to hamstring direct managerial responsibility.

The explosive mixture of growing financial demands, fiscal constraint and bureaucratic rigidity pushed policy-makers across Northern Europe to attempt to develop more flexible organizational frameworks, capable of simultaneously increasing worker participation and improving operating efficiency while also providing a higher standard of patient service. The range of new approaches, either proposed or under trial on a pilot basis, span the spectrum of possibilities, including decentralization and recentralization within the public sector, privatization of service organization and delivery, and a variety of mixed public and private alternatives. As might be anticipated, preferences among these possibilities reflect differences in the history, culture and health system structures in the different countries, as well as in the ideology of their sitting governments.

A similar search for more flexible organizational alternatives is underway in publicly operated health systems beyond Northern

Europe. In Italy, the parliament is expected to adopt legislation which will forge at least minimal links between productivity and individual provider budgets (E. Borgonovi, personal communication, 1989). Further, a new financing arrangement for the national health service has been proposed (Fattore and Garattini, 1989), and a flexible reimbursement experiment has been initiated in the Emilia-Romagna region (Borgonovi, 1990). In Spain, the ministry of health has begun to explore more flexible budgeting arrangements for publicly operated facilities (*Expansion*, 9 March 1990). A national commission to review the structure of the Spanish system was established in autumn 1990 and is expected to present recommendations for major restructuring of service organization and delivery. In Austria, the state of Steiermark has implemented a major reform of its public hospital system, and Vienna's municipal government has under consideration a broad reconstruction of its hospital budgeting arrangements (C. Koeck, personal communication, 1990).

In Eastern Europe, a wide range of organizational experiments of varying character and impact are underway. In Poland, a 1986 ministry of health decision partially linked urban primary care budgets and professional salaries to productivity (Sapinski, 1988). Subsequently, with the rise to power of a Solidarity-led government in 1989, a new health system structure is being designed and is likely to combine national planning and resource allocation with capitation-based GP and case-based hospital reimbursement (Golinowska *et al.*, 1989). In Hungary, a similarly broad reform project is underway, in which national planning and social insurance financing will be combined with efficiency-tied reimbursement of both physicians and hospitals (Sitkery, 1989; Jávor, 1990). In the Soviet Union, expanding upon earlier experiments with production-related salary scales (Ryan, 1987), a radical new model was introduced in three regions in 1988; this assigned hospital budgets to primary care clinics and professional salaries linked to individual and/or team productivity (WHO, 1989). In at least one of these regions – Leningrad – the experiment encountered major difficulties (WHO, 1990). Subsequently, the ministry of health in Moscow has signalled that it may create an entirely new delivery system premised along similar sick-fund insurance lines as those adopted by the emerging systems in Poland and Hungary.

Publicly operated health systems, moreover, are not alone in the search for a more effective structural mix. Pluralist, insurance-based health systems in Europe are developing new mechanisms to reconfigure public and private roles within both their insurance and service delivery sub-sectors (OECD, 1992). In the Netherlands, the health system has come under steady governmental pressure to realign its mix of public and market accountable mechanisms (Rutten, 1986; Lapré, 1988; Saltman and de Roo, 1989). Hybrid models for reform of existing health insurance systems have been put forward in Germany (Finsinger *et al.*, 1986) and in France (Launois *et al.*, 1985). An HMO-based mixed market proposal has been made for Canada (Stoddart and Seldon, 1983), and a variety of mixed-market-based (Enthoven and Kronick, 1989) as well as public-insurance-based (Himmelstein *et al.*, 1989) proposals continue to be put forward in the United States.

The degree of conceptual ferment within pluralist as well as publicly operated health systems, and in Southern, Eastern and Central as well as Northern Europe, suggests that a fundamental shift in the dominant policy paradigm is indeed underway. Moreover, despite statements by conservative governments in countries like the UK and the Netherlands, neo-classical economic models continue to be viewed throughout Europe as a conceptually inappropriate basis for the delivery of essential human services like health care.

When one looks across specifically publicly operated health systems in Northern Europe, the current process of change points in a roughly but discernibly common direction. This convergence focuses on the emergence of what can be termed 'planned markets'. In theoretical terms, this emerging concept of a 'planned market' occupies an intermediate position between command-and-control planning systems, on the one hand, and pure neo-classical market systems, on the other. As presented in Figure 2.1, planned markets

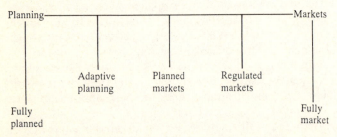

Figure 2.1   The public–private organizational continuum.

are distinct from the 'softer' variants of these two basic paradigms, namely what can be termed 'adaptive' rather than 'fully planned' and 'regulated' rather than 'fully market' organizational frameworks. The differences between the emerging planned market efforts and these other, better known arrangements are instructive.

Adaptive planning, as we use the term, typically involves attempts to decentralize the planning process to smaller bodies located at a lower level in the organizational hierarchy. The actual process of planning itself is unchanged – planners continue to make allocative decisions based on technical criteria and expert knowledge. However, planning takes place further down in the administrative system, where it is presumed to be 'closer' to service providers and, *ipso facto*, more responsive to local requirements. This type of adaptive planning has become quite common throughout the Nordic region; for example, dominating efforts in Sweden to synchronize primary health services more fully with both municipally administered social services and county-run somatic facilities. None the less, in functional terms little, if anything, has changed in the planning process itself.

Regulated markets, on the other side of the organizational continuum, involve the intrusion of state power to limit certain socially or economically disruptive behaviours in a previously existing market system. The state in this model seeks to 'hem in' pre-existing behaviour to limit potential negative consequences. It is a reactive posture, which often fails owing to the inability of regulators to constrain the power of strong privately capitalized companies in established and ongoing markets. Hence, the problem of 'regulatory capture' and other perverse consequences commonly discussed in the political science literature arises.

A 'planned market', in contrast to all four of the above, involves the intentional creation of a new market through the exercise of state power. This market can be consciously designed to achieve state policy objectives through limited and selected use of market instruments. Planned (unlike regulated) markets typically include a substantial number of publicly owned and operated competitors, increasing the leverage of public policy-makers while limiting the impact of the private capital market. Quite unlike adaptive planning, a planned market involves not only the decentralization of the planning process to lower-level administrative entities (or a change in structure) but also the partial replacement of bureaucratic administrative mechanisms with market-derived incentives (a change in function). In contrast to a regulated market, however, a planned market is market-driven only in its mechanisms, not in its operating objective. Regulatory capture is thus more difficult since it would require changes in basic market structure to introduce non-public objectives as formal goals for the market. In effect, the state designs the market before it appears rather than attempting to restrain it after it has run out of control.

The concept behind the term 'planned market' is not entirely new. Publicly operated health systems have previously established more-or-less tightly defined markets in which privately operated providers are encouraged to deliver various peripheral and/or low-intensity services, like dentistry, nursing home and rehabilitation services (McLachlan and Maynard, 1982; SCB, 1988). Similarly, in acute hospitals in the United Kingdom, experimentation with mixed public and private sourcing for non-clinical support services has been underway since the early 1980s (Maynard and Williams, 1984; Key 1988b). Quite new in Northern Europe, however, are attempts to generate explicitly competitive conditions of one type or another inside a wholly publicly capitalized delivery system – what we will term 'public competition'.

In philosophical terms, a strong argument can be made that all markets are by definition political markets, and thus every market is *de facto* a type of planned market (Polanyi, 1944). This theoretical notion, once argued by socialists, now lies at the base of numerous neo-conservative explanations for the social failures experienced in various market sub-sectors (Friedman, 1962), as well as forming the core argument of the 'public choice' school of economics (Buchanan, 1969; Wolf, 1988). The public choice approach, however, goes well beyond earlier socialists, not simply to contend that political markets exist but to insist that they are unnecessary obstacles which distort the economic efficiency of a properly competitive (i.e. theoretically perfect) market.

In the current search for new health care models in Northern Europe, a critical element in defining and monitoring the behaviour of planned markets has been explicitly political in nature. Previous commentators have noted that a range of different market-derived models can be developed, with some suggesting that relative economic merit should be the central criterion for their adoption (Drummond and Maynard, 1988). Beyond specifically economic criteria, however, we believe that the application of market-based incentives to clinical hospital and primary care involves difficult political and normative questions. At the end of the day, the crucial questions to be answered are political and not economic. Publicly responsible authorities must take explicit decisions about the degree of competition to be created, the categories of health sector actors who will compete, the types of incentives to employ, and, most importantly, the new health system objectives to be attained. Public officials are responsible for designing solutions in which perverse social outcomes are foreseen and if at all possible avoided. As one example, the particular type of competition to be introduced can vary along a wide continuum, ranging from the minimal emphasis on internal analysis of production-related information to a no-holds-barred struggle for institutional survival. Given the dynamic character of all forms of competition, public decision-makers are obligated to assess the long-term as well as likely short-term impact of different proposals. Inevitably, these efforts to design hybrid models will reflect important normative choices about the content and character of the values that animate not only the health sector but other public sector human services as well.

In the following three chapters, we explore current efforts to develop planned market models within three Northern European health systems: those of the UK, Sweden and Finland. The three have been selected to illustrate the diversity of present planned market attempts as well as the complexity involved in the design and implementation of these new models. Each of these three countries is in the midst of developing one or more planned market approaches. Although the detailed characteristics of the various models are not yet fully defined, these models and proposals rely upon differing assumptions about the proper mix of public and private roles as well as of market-derived incentive mechanisms in the delivery of clinical services. Taken together, they provide a good picture of the different paths within what is a common political process.

These three countries' divergent planned market models reflect in part the different structures upon which their health systems are based. The British National Health Service has been the archetypal centrally planned, hierarchically managed health care system (Klein, 1983; Harrison, 1988a). Financing comes almost entirely from national tax revenue, and is allocated top-down according to the demographically adjusted RAWP formula among 14 regional and 194 district authorities. Hospital specialists are salaried to the regions, but general practitioners are independent entrepreneurs working for the NHS on a contract basis. The Swedish health system, by contrast, is composed of 26 independent regionally elected (county) health care agencies, which finance two-thirds of their expenditures through their own county tax levied on the personal income of their inhabitants (Saltman, 1988b). The national role is limited to setting broad policy objectives, formulating guidelines and standards, and supplying supplementary funding to support specific national policy objectives (equalizing health resources among the counties, for example). In Sweden both hospital specialists and general practitioners are salaried, and work for the same (county) employer. Finland, to complete this structural triad, has had a nationally planned and half-nationally financed but municipally owned health system, in which hospitals are operated by specific-purpose federations of municipalities (Saltman, 1988a). As in Sweden, general practitioners are employees of relatively large health centres, but general practitioners are municipal employees while hospital specialists are salaried to the municipal federation that operates their hospital.

These three systems also vary considerably on the most widely cited indices for health status and health service resources. Sweden and Finland have substantially better health status indices (lower infant mortality and higher longevity) than does the UK, but they also support a greater number of health-related resources, including physicians and acute hospital beds, per 1000 population.

Beyond these characteristics, the three publicly operated health systems function within quite different political and economic contexts. Politically, the UK has been ruled by a succession of Conservative governments since 1979; Sweden by a Social Democratic regime since 1982; and Finland by a Conservative–Social Democratic coalition since 1987. Economically, per capita income in 1988 was US $21,266 in Sweden, $21,546 in Finland and $14,413 in the UK (OECD: National Accounts).

Despite the structural diversity, each system's relatively high health status outcomes – and for the UK and Finland at relatively low levels of aggregate expenditure – has made it an internationally respected model for publicly operated health systems. The British NHS is often described in health policy literature as the classic centrally budgeted delivery system (Leichter, 1979) and has been an important example to publicly operated systems in Southern Europe as well as in the developing world. The Swedish health care system has been the most visible Nordic system, and is typically viewed as a high quality publicly planned system (Bosworth and Rivlin, 1987; Helco and Madsen, 1987; Ham *et al.*, 1990). The Finnish system, last but not least, was designated a model country system by the World Health Organization in 1982, and has received substantial international attention for its emphasis upon the primary health care sector (Finnish Ministry of Social Affairs and Health, 1987; Pekurinen *et al.*, 1987).

This mix of distinctions and similarities provides a conceptually valuable framework within which to explore these three systems' experiments with various planned market models. Moreover, as suggested in the chapters that follow, health sector politicians and planners in each country are seeking to achieve roughly parallel goals, in the face of essentially equivalent pressures, through divergent and occasionally contradictory policy initiatives. These different strategies, in turn, may generate substantially different long-term outcomes for the structure of health and perhaps public human services generally. As we will examine below, the diversity of mechanisms which can be employed to create a planned market suggests that the decision to adopt a hybrid public–private health system solution may well signal only the beginning rather than the end of the most important internal policy debate.

3

PLANNING AND MARKETS IN THE UNITED KINGDOM

THE POLICY CONTEXT

The United Kingdom provides a case study in the complex process of introducing planned market mechanisms into a command-and-control health system. On the one hand, the intellectual and political pressures in support of substantial change have been stronger in the UK than in any other Northern European country. Yet on the other hand, the central defining characteristic of the actual reform process, once it got underway some ten years into Conservative Party rule, has been a pronounced hesitancy to push announced proposals through to completion. By spring 1991, a reform package which had initially emphasized multiple market-style mechanisms, including a mixed public/private market for service provision, had been scaled back to a considerably less radical framework within which most market initiatives will be, as the *Economist* (9 February 1991, pp. 61–2) described it, 'tightly controlled from the centre'.

The debate concerning market approaches versus planning approaches to health care in the United Kingdom has reflected the political pre-eminence of the Conservative Party throughout the 1980s. Given that the national government actively sought to cultivate an entrepreneurial orientation within all sectors of British society, it was somewhat surprising that the British National Health Service (NHS) – a centrally planned agency providing universal access free of charge at the point of service – had escaped most of the decade relatively unscathed (Maxwell, 1988). This special status continued despite the build-up of internal pressures in the NHS created by a combination of tightly constrained operating budgets

(Higgins, 1988), continued capital starvation and lengthening patient queues for elective procedures (Yates, 1987), as well as, externally, the growing strength of a renascent private sector (Ascher, 1987; Higgins, 1988). Until 1989, the government limited itself to ameliorative structural changes in the existing command-and-control planning structure, most notably at district health authority level with the 1983 replacement of consensus-based decision-making by corporate-style 'general management' (Harrison, 1988b).

The debate over alternative financing and delivery systems intensified as the long-term liabilities of the existing NHS structure became increasingly evident (Ham *et al.,* 1990). In 1985, a proposal by an American economist to transform the NHS into a somewhat misnamed 'internal market', including private as well as public providers (Enthoven, 1985), attracted widespread attention. The flow of reform proposals expanded once the Prime Minister, in January 1988, seized upon fiscal turmoil in the health sector as justification for a ministerial review of the NHS. Numerous academics (Bevan, 1989; Bevan and Marinker, 1989) and organizations (Institute for Health Service Management, 1988) developed their own market-influenced proposals to compete with more explicit market-driven models put forward by right-wing think tanks like the Adam Smith Institute (Butler and Pirie, 1988) and the Centre for Policy Studies (Goldsmith and Willetts, 1988). This debate sharpened the clash between cautious reformers, who preferred to adopt market-generated incentives in carefully calibrated doses, and radical marketeers who called for the replacement of the NHS with an insurance-based variant of the United States health system.

The intellectual evolution of the year-long ministerial review itself provides an instructive story about the complexity of generating structural change within a large publicly operated health system. Although initially there was considerable sympathy for replacing the NHS with a pluralist system based on private health insurance (perhaps along the lines of the then West German framework), these ideas steadily lost ground to less Conservatively correct but more clinically, administratively and – most important of all – financially practical alternatives which maintained a substantial degree of central government control over expenditures.

The final proposal, as presented in the 1989 white paper entitled

Working for Patients, cobbled together a compromise solution in which a variety of market-oriented initiatives would be superimposed upon the existing top-down administrative structure. This approach had a certain political attractiveness, in that the government could defend the review's outcome as radically new (to its own right wing) yet protective of traditional NHS values (to the general population). Using the terminology developed in Chapter 1, the Prime Minister could hail the outcome to the first audience as a strategic reform, which would generate thoroughgoing change at every level of the health service, while simultaneously insisting to the wider public that the white paper was no more than a reformist reform, which would preserve the essential core of the NHS for the future.

Whatever the government's true intentions might have been, the time since the presentation of the white paper has seen continual back-tracking from the more radical or strategic reform elements of the programme. At the point of actual implementation in April 1991 (following the adoption of the NHS and Community Care Act in July 1990), the white paper's market-oriented mechanisms had been largely neutralized or postponed indefinitely. The planned market model being introduced in the UK – at least for year 1 as part of the so-called 'smooth take-off' – is substantially less dependent upon market mechanisms (mixed private and public contracting for services; managerial autonomy for opted-out hospitals) than was the original white paper model. As the *Economist*'s comment implies, the planned market model to be implemented more than three years after the commencement of Mrs Thatcher's ministerial review is decidedly less dramatic than that envisioned either at the beginning of the process in 1988 or from the compromise proposal contained in the 1989 white paper.

In this chapter we explore the development of a planned market model in the UK from two key perspectives. First, we briefly review three precursor reforms or reform proposals which provided the political and administrative context for the 1988 ministerial review. These were the 1983 introduction of general management into the NHS, the simultaneous introduction of performance indicators and clinical budgeting for specialist physicians, and the 1988 Griffith Report on restructuring community care. Second, we examine the white paper proposals themselves, and compare them with the rather different planned market model that was implemented in April 1991.

THREE PRECURSOR INNOVATIONS

The introduction of general management

In June 1984, the UK government announced that it would 'fully implement' the reform proposals for the NHS contained within the October 1983 Griffiths Report. These proposals called for a full-time NHS management board at the national level, and for the replacement of the then current system of team-based consensus management by a more business-like system of regional, district and unit 'general managers'. Reflecting the private sector perspective of the report's senior author, Roy Griffiths, managing director of the Sainsbury's supermarket chain, this shift in management structure was intended to create conditions for more flexible, entrepreneurial decision-making at the operating authority level. As part of the effort to encourage entrepreneurial behaviour, general managers were to be hired on short-term contracts that would be subject to performance appraisal before renewal. The stated objective in making this change was to achieve increased efficiency and value for money within the NHS. By autumn 1985, two years after the Griffiths Report was published, general managers were in place throughout the NHS (Parston, 1988).

This attempt to create private sector style managers inside the health service met with only limited success. The process of adaptation within the NHS, which had an inbred culture that emphasized organizational stability (some might say bureaucratic inertia), was uneven and occasionally uncomfortable. The inadequacy of existing information and accounting systems reduced the new managers' degrees of freedom, and specialist physicians continued to dominate hospital decision-making processes (Harrison *et al.*, 1989b). More fundamentally, the central intention of generating managerial initiative at the local level tended to contradict the purpose of maintaining a centrally structured, tightly budgeted national service in the first place (Birch and Maynard, 1988; Key, 1988b).

If one evaluates this shift in decision-making structure at the operating authority level exclusively on its own terms, Griffiths's general managers become a classic example of 'reformist reform': Griffiths was simply restructuring the command-and-control process within the state bureaucracy for health (Strong and Robinson, 1990). The fact that the particular concept adopted – individually responsible managers – was at the time associated more with private than with public sector management in the United Kingdom did not alter the centralized planning framework within which the new personnel were placed. From this perspective, the Griffiths framework clarified the underlying Weberian organizational principle upon which NHS decision-making continued to be based. The simultaneous adoption of additional private sector style mechanisms, such as performance indicators for hospitals and specialist physicians, authority to contract out for ancillary services and certain liberalized controls (in theory if not practice) over capital (Key, 1988b) and estate management (Wickings and Child, 1988), can be viewed as confirmation of a strategy which placed private sector mechanisms in service to a command-and-control budgeting and reporting process.

One comes to a different assessment of general management if one views the Griffiths reforms in a broader perspective that includes the January 1989 white paper and likely changes during the 1990s. The introduction of general management becomes very much a 'strategic reform', in that it was a necessary step in creating the preconditions for an eventual shift from a tightly planned 'administered' system to a competition-driven 'managed' delivery structure. In this view, the January 1989 white paper served to confirm the long-range mission of general management as a mechanism through which decision-making autonomy and entrepreneurial initiative at the unit and district level could be introduced.

This 'strategic' interpretation of the general management reform is strengthened by the emphasis in both the 1983 Griffiths Report and the 1989 white paper upon local managerial autonomy in contradistinction to, indeed in direct opposition to, formal municipal or community participation in health service decisions. A negative view of municipal participation was a consistent characteristic of the Thatcher government, as reflected in a variety of efforts to strip local government of authority and revenue (Hood, 1988). The 1989 white paper further reduced the vestigial role of municipal and local community participation in health service decision-making in two respects. First, local authorities (Britain's municipal governments) would lose their seats on district health authorities. Second, the white paper pushed district health authorities to adopt a private sector management style in which narrow 'business' criteria were to predominate over the community-level concerns that local authority members had typically raised.

If one pursues this second, 'strategic reform' interpretation of the 1983 Griffiths proposals, the question of introducing general management can be viewed as an issue of creating 'planned markets'. The general management reform became a cornerstone in the British government's emerging effort to generate entrepreneurial flexibility at the operating level within a globally budgeted and politically constrained national health system.

Performance indicators and management budgeting

Concurrent with the introduction of general management, the 1983 Griffiths Report supported the adoption of more sophisticated managerial techniques at the district health authority and operating unit (mainly hospital) levels. The stated objective was to facilitate a closer correspondence between the budget allocated to clinical units and the work performed by professional providers. The proposed mechanism for closer scrutiny of provider performance was the recently developed system of 'performance indicators', while the instrument selected to incorporate provider professionals – most specifically hospital specialists – into the managerial process was to be 'management budgeting'.

The concept of performance indicators involved the generation of comparable statistics on service outputs and resource consumption broken down into functional categories: clinical activity, manpower, finance and estate management (Birch and Maynard, 1988). Their purpose was not to provide the basis for specific decisions but rather to be an informational warning system which could identify potential problem areas for further investigation. The intention was that general managers would respond to these distress signals with more detailed productivity evaluation.

The concept of management budgeting was first tested in a pilot programme involving six sites in 1986 (four in acute units; two for community services) with the intention of generalizing the results, if successful, to acute units in all districts by 1992 (Coles, 1988). Now labelled 'resource management', the initiative has the central purpose of involving hospital specialists in the management of their clinical units. Like similar efforts in the United States (Zuidema, 1980) and Sweden (Saltman, 1986), the concept is that medical specialists help to select and then enforce clinical limitations necessary to achieve maximum benefit from a fixed level of funding. In effect, since specialists authorize an overwhelming proportion of hospital expenditures, one way to increase value for money is to harness these physicians to the achievement of explicitly managerial goals.

The results from both initiatives were widely characterized as disappointing (Ham and Hunter, 1988). The performance indicators generated overly simplistic data since they were not adjusted for case mix or other structural variations among districts, nor were they linked to the quality of outcomes obtained (Birch and Maynard, 1988). Moreover, rather than simply providing warning signals, the data generated were used directly for managerial decision-making, particularly to identify areas for cutbacks to achieve nationally and/or regionally mandated cost reductions. In effect, unadjusted raw data were used not to improve management efficiency but to cut back levels of service.

Management budgeting, similarly, suffered in the acute trial locations from the inadequate quality of the information generated, as well as from a lack of systematic attention from a senior staff preoccupied with the implementation of general management (Coles, 1988). Moreover, the tight time scale for introduction resulted in a financially oriented – rather than clinically and/or outcome oriented – information system. While the demonstration generated increasing willingness on the part of hospital specialists to enter into resource-related discussions, the dominant interest of the NHS management board in improved financial results could well dissuade physicians from future participation.

From the perspective of constructing planned markets, both the performance indicator and the management budgeting initiatives sought to introduce more appropriate management information systems into existing NHS decision-making processes. In the sense that good production-related cost information is an essential precondition to making more efficient operating decisions, both initiatives can be seen as narrowly reflecting market-related incentives to improve overall organizational productivity and hence value for money. Neither initiative, however, was implemented in a broader managerial context which incorporated adequate market-related objectives or behaviour. Neither information system was related back to the district's annual budget allocation, so as to tie information about productivity to concurrent decisions about annual expenditures. Although general managers were on short-term contracts subject to performance appraisal, their own annual salaries were only indirectly linked to the districts' overall performance as indicated on either information system. Hospital specialists were not subject to performance appraisal and they did not have performance-linked salaries.

In sum, while the overall information system concept was adopted from the private sector, it was introduced into an organizational decision-making environment that remained hierarchical in both structure and function. The necessary linkage between appropriating the *form* from the private sector and taking essential market-driven *content* as it affects decision-making and resource allocation had not yet been made. As a consequence, although these two initiatives presaged subsequent efforts to utilize market-generated mechanisms to obtain a strategically intended outcome, they were not designed as elements of a planned market strategy.

Restructuring community service

The third precursor to the 1989 white paper was the community care proposal put forward in 1988. In its presentation of a mixed market of service providers, including private for-profit and private not-for-profit (or voluntary) as well as publicly operated institutions, the 1988 community care report sketched out a conceptual framework which would be extended one year later to the entire health service. Although only a proposal rather than an actual reform, this community care report may well have rivalled the introduction of general management as a forebear of the 1989 white paper.

The reorganization of community care has been a topic of debate in the UK at least since a 1976 ministry report recognized the importance of expanding home care services (Wistow, 1988). Subsequently, two new financial mechanisms were superimposed upon the joint NHS–local authority consultative committees which remained the basic mechanism for achieving a coordinated health and social service policy. One, termed 'joint finance', began in the late 1970s and a second programme, known as 'resource transfers' or 'care in the community', began in 1983 and initially allowed health authorities to commit NHS funds to local authorities for three years (later extended). Neither programme, however, was particularly successful (Wistow, 1988). A central limitation was that their funds had to be 'top-sliced' from existing NHS allocations, so that they were always underfunded. Moreover, in the joint finance programme, there was no assurance that municipal authorities would allocate health service funds to address the issue of greatest concern to the NHS, which was the question of 'bed-blockers' who were waiting for community placement.

The 1988 Griffiths Report, *Community Care: Agenda for Action*, proposed replacing collaborative planning techniques with a market-based set of organizational mechanisms and solutions. The report proposed that local authorities be held responsible only 'to ensure that care is provided', with the actual service delivery to be determined via competitive tenders and contracts with both public institutions and various for-profit and not-for-profit private sector companies (HMSO, 1988, p. vii). The report followed the logic of public finance for private provision further by suggesting that local authorities should create voucher systems to allow patients to choose among different providers, and in so doing seek to 'maximize choice and competition' (HMSO, 1988, p. 15).

Beyond advocating this mixed economy for social service delivery, the report said little about resolving the complicated problem of integration between health and social service authorities. The major exception was to suggest that health and social service agencies review each other's plans (HMSO, 1988, p. 16). Thus, while this report contained planned market elements, the scope of these changes was limited to services within the social service sector, and little provision was made to accommodate the contradictory mix of intra-sector market and extra-sector planning mechanisms.

THE 1989 WHITE PAPER

The release in January 1989 of *Working for Patients* (HMSO, 1989), which summarized the policy proposals reached by the government's ministerial review of the National Health Service, brought the decade-long British debate over the future of the NHS to a critical juncture. Building upon earlier suggestions to create an 'internal market' (Enthoven, 1985) or a 'provider market' (Institute for Health Service Management, 1988), as well as the 1988 Griffiths proposals for community care (HMSO, 1988), the government proposed to establish a mixed public/private market for the provision of health services, accountable to district health authorities which would be responsible for running this new market on a bid and contract basis. While tax-based finance of the health service was to be retained, a variety of market mechanisms were to be adopted as the means to achieve central government's objectives. Although its content reflected political compromise, the white paper's intention was none the less to steer Britain's publicly operated health service directly into as yet uncharted planned market waters.

The Conservative government sought to attain its entrepreneurial objectives by the introduction of three major structural changes in the organization of the NHS. First, the role of the district health authority would undergo a fundamental shift. District authorities would continue to receive a centrally allocated public budget but would no longer be the sole providers of services. Instead, the district authority would be transformed into a purchasing agent, seeking care for patients from multiple sources, including publicly operated institutions within its own district, publicly operated institutions in other districts elsewhere in the UK, private not-for-profit and/or for-profit institutions, and possibly new public–private joint ventures. The language of the white paper insisted that the district authorities should pursue diverse providers: 'In future, each DHA's duty would be to buy the best service it can from its own hospital, from other authorities' hospitals, from self-governing hospitals or from the private sector' (HMSO, 1989, p. 33). The white paper subsequently adopted Enthoven's language in explanation of how the government defined 'best' in the above statement of principle:

> Health authorities carrying out their new role as purchasers rather than providers of care will buy in services from the private sector if it offers *a better deal* than is available from NHS hospitals (emphasis added).
>
> (HMSO, 1989, p. 68)

The second major change put forward by the white paper was that larger acute hospitals would be encouraged to 'opt out' of the service, becoming 'self-governing' institutions under the authority of an independent non-profit trust. In much the same manner as an independent general hospital in pluralist health systems like those of the Netherlands or the United States, each independent acute institution would be expected to obtain patients by selling its services – presumably on quality as well as cost – to various district health authorities but also to privately insured and potentially foreign-insured patients as well. Self-governing hospitals would be entitled to have contracts directly with all their staff, including hospital specialists, and full control over their operating and capital decisions. The only requirements placed on these hospitals in the 1989 white paper were that they have in place a medical audit system before opting out of the health service and that they continue to provide essential core services like accident and emergency if no alternative source of care existed.

The third major structural change involved giving large general practitioner (GP) group practices control over part of their patients' annual acute care hospital budget. Eligible practices should have over 11 000 enrolled patients, double the national average, which amounted to some 9 per cent of all GP practices and covered about 25 per cent of the total population (HMSO, 1989, p. 50) (this figure was subsequently reduced to 9000 patients). Beyond primary care and prescription services (which would be cash-limited for the first time since the NHS started), these new 'practice budgets' would include certain selected outpatient, inpatient and diagnostic services. The stated intention was to encourage the GP to negotiate 'fixed-price contracts for each speciality', sending patients to whatever publicly operated, not-for-profit or for-profit hospital offered 'the best deals' (HMSO, 1989, p. 52). The centrality of financial motivation for the government also emerged in detailed suggestions such as the following: 'Practices will want to hold some money back, to keep open the possibility of obtaining services at marginal cost where hospitals have spare capacity to offer in the course of the year' (HMSO, 1989, p. 52).

The white paper further proposes various managerial mechanisms to encourage fund-holding practices to engage in prudent referral and purchasing behaviour. For instance, practices will be allowed to overspend by up to 5 per cent 'for good clinical reasons', but the overspend is to be repaid the following year. Another example, adopted from certain health maintenance organizations in the United States, would allow GPs to retain a significant proportion of their practice savings to be spent as they wish.

As these three major changes suggest, the white paper proposals would transform the 40-year-old NHS from the archetypal centrally planned health system into the most thoroughly mixed market in Northern Europe. After implementation, the remaining top-down administrative system would concern itself predominantly with budgetary and fiscal matters, while the delivery of services would increasingly devolve to more-or-less autonomous, overlapping and competing units of diverse ownership characteristics. General managers in the public sector at hospital, district authority and ultimately budget-holding GP practice levels would be encouraged to adopt managerial techniques closely associated with private business – most specifically, contracting patient care out to providers offering 'the best deal'. Finally, while patients would be given greater opportunity to change their general practitioners, they would be likely to find themselves obligated to obtain ambulatory and inpatient hospital care in accordance with contracts negotiated by the district health authority or a budget-holding GP practice.

Viewed more broadly, the white paper proposals clearly de-emphasize direct democratic participation in health-related decision-making. Beyond restrictions on patient choice of hospital provider (Green *et al.*, 1990), the proposed planned market intentionally downgrades the influence of local authority or community level officials, and thus adopts almost exclusively financial (as against political or participatory) criteria for goal-setting and achievement. Further, the market structure defined in *Working for Patients* focused predominantly upon district authority and acute hospitals – with an internally competing proposal based upon GP practices contracting for certain hospital services – to the detriment of preventive, intra-sectoral (particularly hospital and social service) and inter-sectoral (educational, housing, job training, day care, etc.) matters (Harrison *et al.*, 1989a).

Two additional aspects of the white paper proposals have been the subject of considerable dispute. One has been the clear intention to introduce a mixed public and private market for the provision of services, through contracts to be negotiated with private for-profit as well as other public institutions. From the perspective of white paper proponents, the adoption of this new *modus operandi* as well as a willingness to work with private for-profit providers would enable the public system to adopt the flexibility and efficiency of the private sector. Responding to the decade-long growth of the private health sector in the UK (Higgins, 1988), and also capitalizing on the introduction of district and unit general managers in the mid-1980s, this view describes the NHS as learning useful managerial lessons from the private sector. Moreover, the set of relationships likely to evolve between the publicly operated and private for-profit and not-for-profit providers is characterized as complementary and supportive.

Critics of the white paper proposals tend to see the emerging relations between public and private sectors in quite another light.

They fear that publicly operated units, in order to compete for contracts with for-profit providers, will find themselves forced to jettison components of their present treatment patterns which private sector competitors do not offer – for example, educating patients about their condition, or providing social services to less-well-off or otherwise vulnerable patients. The result, critics suggest, is that public hospitals in the UK ultimately would follow mission-oriented not-for-profit hospitals in the USA (Gray, 1986) in remaking themselves in the image of their for-profit counter-parts, to the detriment of public service objectives.

A second point of contention in the white paper proposals concerns the likely impact upon the ability of patients to influence where and under what conditions they receive care. Mrs Thatcher argued in her foreword that 'All the proposals in this white paper put the needs of patients first' (HMSO, 1989). With the exception of an explicit promise (without specifics) to make it easier for patients to change GP lists, the basis of the government's argument appeared to be the neo-classical economic notion that, with the mixed market's presumed increase in operating efficiency, more services would be available to enable patients to be treated more rapidly.

Critics of this mixed market approach view the central thrust of the white paper as empowering managers within district authorities or budget-holding general practices, who would be able to channel patients towards providers that met contract requirements tied closely to issues of price. Patients, in this view, would have even less influence in this new contract-based arrangement than they had under the previous command-and-control model (Green *et al.*, 1990). Moreover, the assumption that patient selection of GP carries with it a full and sufficient exercise of patient sovereignty – that patients ought not to be able to influence the site of hospital treatment or the specialists who deliver it – transcends even the limitations on patient choice that have emerged in the USA with the development of health maintenance organizations (HMOs), and preferred provider organizations (PPOs).

IMPLEMENTATION AND FUTURE POLICY

The initial schedule for implementation of the white paper's planned market proposals called for full-scale introduction of a mixed market in April 1991. As noted in the chapter introduction, this optimistic scenario was derailed by a combination of logistical, political and most of all substantive problems with the white paper proposals.

First, logistically, the government appeared to have under-estimated the sheer magnitude of an effort to re-shape a million-employee organization that serves a population of more than 50 million people. Despite the earlier introduction of general manage-ment, it was apparent by summer 1990 that a number of the 14 British NHS regions lacked the necessary managerial skills to take the mixed market model forward in the near term. Additional difficulties were caused by the lack of fit between the new expectations for personnel activities and the organizational culture of the NHS, and by the strong and publicly advertised opposition of the British Medical Association. With the exception of managers in some of the larger hospitals likely to become self-governing trusts, there was little enthusiasm for the reforms from inside the health service, which further burdened the government's ambitious sched-ule for implementation.

Second, politically, the Conservative Party feared that the unpopularity of the proposed NHS reforms would further weaken its standing in the polls, potentially jeopardizing its chances of re-election in the national balloting to be called by June 1992. By late 1990 there was also clear evidence that administrative and budgetary preparations for the introduction of the reform model would result in a further lengthening of the NHS waiting lists for elective procedures. Despite the expenditure of £120 million (US $200 million) over the previous four years on special initiatives to cut waiting times, by winter 1990–1 these lists approached the one million mark for England alone – a threshold that Conservative ministers had set as a political danger point (*Guardian Weekly*, 3 February, 1991). A key contributing factor to this lengthening of waiting lists was the intention of government ministers to hold district authorities to their budgets so as to clear the books for the introduction of the new mixed market arrangements. Further, the prospect of allowing opted-out hospitals to borrow private capital for unrestricted expansion seemed increasingly at odds with the government's overall macroeconomic policy of reducing public sector expenditures.

Third, substantively, there appeared to be growing misgivings about the mixed market focus of the white paper proposals themselves, and about the need for pilot and demonstration projects before full-scale implementation (Robinson, 1988). A test simulation of the model conducted in May 1990, dubbed the 'rubber windmill' experiment, produced a market crash which led some observers to conclude that more design work was necessary. Other observers, noting the introduction of intentional misinformation by some participants in the rubber windmill's contract negotiations, as well as the rapidity with which participants forgot the concerns of patients, concluded that a contract-based planned market would inevitably short-change patient interests.

Taken together, these logistical, political and substantive concerns led to a decision by the Conservative government to pull back from the most aggressively market-oriented aspects of the white paper proposals. In an attempt to ensure a 'smooth take-off' with 'no surprises', the government withdrew two key elements of the original proposals. First, district authorities will not switch over to negotiated contracts to obtain services from public providers, and there will be no new contracts with private providers for at least the first year. Instead, district revenue will flow exactly as it has in the past, on a resource input rather than a performance output basis, to be termed 'block contracting'. Second, self-governing hospital trusts (of which 57 were to be established in 1991) will lose several key levers of their anticipated managerial autonomy. They will have to have capital expenditures approved by the Treasury Department at central government, which will force hospitals to compete with each other for permission. They also will be required to pay their junior physicians at nationally negotiated rates (*Economist*, 9 February 1991, pp. 61–2).

These two changes in the reform proposal would appear effectively to stymie the creation of either a mixed public/private market or entrepreneurial district authorities and hospitals. The effect clearly will be to squeeze the proposed planned market down to its irreducible minimum of fund-holding general practices. This outcome is intriguing in that this is the component of the white paper proposals that *fuses* finance and provision together in a single set of administrative hands, unlike the district authority and hospital proposals, which sought exactly the opposite result of *separating* finance from service provision. Moreover, from an international perspective the remaining fund-holding general practice format appears to resemble the essence of the HMO approach in the United States. It remains to be seen whether the British approach will generate the various acquired diseases often attributed to HMOs: adverse selection, undertreatment of poor and chronically ill patients, and an uneasiness in taking financial responsibility for elderly patients. There is some speculation that the British model will allow substantial jockeying for advantage between fund-holding and non-fund-holding GPs, not least with regard to the costs of hospital care contracted for by district health authorities.

Whatever the outcome of the current government's efforts to restructure the NHS, over the longer term the health service is likely to continue to decentralize increasing aspects of operating control to professional providers and provider units. The several processes detailed above suggest that in the UK, as elsewhere, the daily struggle for control over budgets and institutions will continue to be fought out between administration, in the modern guise of general managers, and practising physicians. By devolving operating control to the institutional level, the character of the struggle may shift but the essential complexities involved in managing physician practice patterns will continue to dominate organizational decision-making. As the NHS gropes towards a specifically British form of planned market – be it a neo-classically influenced mixed market or something else – the complications of adapting private sector incentives to public sector objectives also will remain. British political culture, despite a generation of the welfare state, remains individualistic at its core and hence more responsive to market types of thinking than are Nordic societies with their more collectivist philosophical roots. However, the challenge of coupling preventive to curative care, or hospital to home care, confronts all publicly operated health systems in the 1990s, and the degree of success achieved by specifically British planned market models will be closely scrutinized.

4

PLANNING AND MARKETS IN SWEDEN

THE POLICY CONTEXT

Present policy debate in Sweden signals important changes in the long-term development of its health care system. In a major break with past approaches, it has become likely that planned market initiatives will be incorporated within that development process, coupled to a continued decentralization of administrative responsibility to county and/or municipal level governments. Conversely, in part as a consequence of thoroughgoing decentralization, there is growing discussion about the long-term policy consequences that may accompany regional or local administrative independence. The growing operational autonomy of the 26 county councils, as expressed in present experiments with various planned market models, has underscored questions about the ability of the national government to attain major normative and fiscal objectives. Although administrative decentralization is deeply rooted within official public sector objectives, local autonomy could undercut national commitments to, for example, guarantee equal access to services or reduce total public sector expenditures.

This debate over appropriate levels and mechanisms of health sector accountability reflects two fundamental shifts in the underlying policy context. First, the national government faces strong internal and external pressures to restrain overall public expenditures, particularly in human services like health care. Internal pressures include the perceived importance of reducing income tax rates to stimulate greater individual productivity – a particular problem given Sweden's relatively high marginal tax rates and relatively low current rate of economic growth. External pressures include the emerging single European market in 1992, the expected Swedish application for membership in the European Community, and the necessity of aligning Swedish economic policy to that of its major trading partners if Swedish companies are to remain internationally competitive.

A second fundamental shift in the policy context, which only partially reflects economic pressures, is the increased awareness among most Swedish policy-makers of the limitations of traditional health planning models (Lundberg, 1985). At the national political level, government officials have become increasingly uncomfortable with command-and-control planning approaches as a basis for problem solving. At the county council administrative level, where operating decisions must be taken and defended, there is growing recognition that strictly allocative models are not well suited to making the difficult service trade-offs that health providers continue to confront.

The perception in Sweden of the inadequacy of traditional planning models has been related more to the processes than to the objectives of these models. A particular concern has been the apparent disjuncture between a rapid rate of change in the external clinical and social environment and a slow rate of health sector response. Among other difficulties, this organizational sluggishness helped to create waiting periods of up to two years for certain elective surgical procedures. These queues became a source of growing embarrassment for the health system (Heister and Gustavsson, 1989; *Svenska Dagbladet*, 7 August 1989) and the national Social Democratic government. Although health officials preferred to blame non-planning factors such as changes in clinical procedures and indications, the Ministry of Health's 1987 decision to invest 70 million crowns to reduce queues for intra-ocular lens implants, full hip replacements and coronary by-pass procedures (Socialstyrelsen, 1988) suggests that a key problem was a lack of organizational prioritization and political will.

Problems caused by the lugubrious nature of the health planning process have been compounded by the tendency of short-term planned solutions to generate longer-term problems somewhere else in the delivery system. For example, the 'success' of the county planning apparatus in the early 1980s in reducing aggregate expenditures by reducing growth in wages to personnel helped to bring about the 'failure' of the planning process in the late 1980s, when this lower wage scale restricted the counties' ability to attract needed nursing and home care personnel. In a similar pattern, the earlier emphasis of health planners upon expanding primary care services, which required a simultaneous downgrading of the (then overbuilt) hospital sector, helped to generate renewed pressures from 1987 to reprioritize resources for intensive hospital services. One can also point to increased efforts to control expenditures in county-funded hospital clinics, which have led to conflicts with municipally funded social services over issues of principle as well as over individual cases.

The planning dilemmas faced by the Swedish counties in the 1980s resemble the internal organizational problems which afflicted large private sector corporations in the 1950s and 1960s, and which gave rise to contingency theory (Neuhauser, 1986). Faced with a complex multi-division structure and a rapidly changing external environment, the successful organization would, according to contingency theorists, differentiate its internal management processes while simultaneously pursuing a set of integrated strategic objectives (Lawrence and Lorsch, 1969). The difficulties of the planning process in the Swedish health sector, from this perspective, reflect the insensitivity of traditional allocative planning mechanisms to a shifting clinical, popular and political environment. Despite expectations that 1983 legislation which decentralized administrative authority to the 26 counties would generate a 'service culture' rather than an 'agency culture', despite further intra-county decentralization to hospital and primary care subdistricts in pursuit of the same objective, the traditional health planning model has proved to be too congenitally linear in its internal logic to respond adequately. One national official described the Swedish counties' current dilemma as one in which 'we must plan, but we must plan for flexibility'. Another official summarized the new policy challenge in Sweden with the following formula: 'the emphasis must be on equity of value not of form.'

In part as a consequence of reduced faith in the county-based planning system, there is renewed interest at the national and municipal levels in expanding their roles in, respectively, health policy and service delivery areas. At the national level, there is a wide-ranging debate over the proper locus of national health policy formulation. This is a relatively new discussion in Sweden (Ham *et al.*, 1990) in which national officials have begun to question whether the national government has allowed too much policy as well as administrative responsibility to devolve to the county councils. The sharp framing of this debate by one Swedish official – 'Sweden is not a federation of county councils, it's one national state, and it should have one national health policy' – is echoed by several recent national policy mechanisms: the national queue initiative (now dropped), a national health and medical care committee chaired by the prime minister, and a new ministry unit for technology assessment. A further reflection of this debate can be found in contingency planning by the Federation of County Councils to widen its organizational focus to emphasize its 'regional planning' function (Landstingsförbundet, 1986). This national versus county struggle is tempered by the fact that both levels of government are led by Social Democratic politicians, a point which supports the argument that the problem has been viewed as largely structural rather than ideological in character. In spring 1990 a national investigatory commission was established to explore future organizational alternatives for the Swedish health system, called the 'Crossroads Project'. The commission's brief was to provide a set of possible scenarios for consideration by the three national organizations that set the project up: the Federation of County Councils, the National Board of Health and Welfare, and the Ministry of Social Affairs and Health. A final report was presented to the June 1991 congress of the Federation of County Councils.

A second, municipally driven debate concerns the long-term efficiency and effectiveness of keeping primary health and primary medical services within the existing county council system, rather than consolidating them with social services under the overall supervision of the municipalities. This issue has a long history, and it re-emerged in a 1989 proposal by the ministry to the parliament to give municipalities final responsibility for all services received by the elderly (Landstingsförbundet, 1989).

A third policy debate concerns the consolidation of two independent work-related funding arrangements into what would be a single integrated health sector financing structure (Finansdepartmentet, 1987). There is broad discussion as to whether one of these arrangements, the national sickness payment mechanism, should be directly linked with the health systems, to enable sickness payments to be diverted where appropriate to finance more rapid delivery of curative and rehabilitative services. This would speed both the treatment and the return to work of many individuals who currently draw lengthy sickness payments and often take early retirement. A similar set of concerns revolves around the second work-related arrangement, workers' compensation insurance, particularly in the area of rehabilitative services.

While all three of these ongoing debates suggest the degree to which Swedish health policy is under review, they do not fully convey the scope of the current process of change. In the following section on structural innovations, the breadth of this process, and the role of both planned market and public firms that is emerging within it, are sketched out in more detail.

RECENT STRUCTURAL INNOVATIONS

The Dagmar Reform

A major Swedish initiative in the area of planned markets is the Dagmar Reform of 1985, which restructured national health insurance payments for ambulatory physician visits. Nominally, it was designed to reinforce existing long-term policy objectives by consolidating all primary care services into the publicly operated county health system. In practice, it established 26 separate county-led planned markets for ambulatory care services, several of which soon developed in rather different policy directions.

A central connecting thread of recent Swedish health policy has been its emphasis upon developing primary and preventive health services within the publicly operated health system. This policy line can be traced back to the Höjer Report of 1948 (named for the highly respected but politically controversial head of the National Board of Health during the 1940s) which argued for the establishment of a new publicly operated system of health centres that could ensure the provision of comprehensive preventive as well as curative medical services to all Swedish citizens (Serner, 1980). Although Höjer's proposals initially attracted support only in the labour movement, they have come to form the core of Swedish health policy for more than a generation (Saltman, 1988b).

In organizational terms, the Höjer Report stimulated a two-part policy evolution in which Swedish health and medical activities were increasingly concentrated (generally by means of decentralization from national bodies) in the county councils and, equally importantly, delivery of clinical services increasingly became a public sector responsibility. This policy ran from the 1955 implementation of universal health insurance for ambulatory care (which introduced publicly set ceilings for insurance reimbursement to general practitioners), the 1959 end of pay-beds in county hospitals and the 1963 transfer to the counties of the state-run system of district medical officers, through to the 1970 Seven Crown Reform that ended most private ambulatory care by publicly employed hospital specialists, and the parliamentary acts of 1973 and 1983.

From this historical perspective, the Dagmar Reform of 1985 fulfilled a dual role. On the one hand, it was the capstone in the creation of a primary-care-based, county council operated health system. On the other hand, however, the Dagmar Reform began the unravelling of national planning policy, facilitating the emergence of planned markets and organizational pluralism as the dominant policy perspective in the late 1980s.

The central purpose of the Dagmar Reform was to consolidate the county councils' planning authority over ambulatory physician visits. This was to be accomplished through two changes in the way in which national health insurance reimbursed providers for ambulatory visits. First, the prior fee-for-service mechanism was restructured into an annual capitated (age and sex adjusted) payment. Second, all capitated payments were made directly to the county councils, which then were responsible for determining which (if any) funds, and on what basis, should be made available to fund private practitioners. In addition, it was anticipated that the newly centralized funding mechanism would assist counties in attracting physicians to more rural districts of the country. Dagmar effectively reinforced the official responsibility for health services given to the counties under the 1983 Health Act. By channelling all ambulatory care insurance funds through the county councils on a capitated basis, Dagmar enabled the counties to plan annual fixed budgets for primary services as well as to take full demographic responsibility. In these two respects, Dagmar fitted well with the broad planning thrust of standard post-Höjer health policy.

This financial restructuring has also had important implications for the public–private mix in ambulatory care. Private practitioners continue to deliver publicly insured visits only with the explicit permission of, and only up to the volume agreed by, the county council. Thus, with the consolidation of planning and financing responsibility for primary care in county hands, the private sector became fully dependent on the public sector for its survival. Interpreted in the light of mainstream Swedish health policy, this too appears to fulfil the planning model's long-held promise of a fully public ambulatory service.

In practice, the implementation of the Dagmar Reform produced a variegated outcome. Reflecting recent shifts in underlying political, social and clinical conditions, including their decision-making independence, different counties selected different strategies. Some county councils did seize upon the Dagmar mechanism to restrict the total volume of private visits, and also to reduce the total number of private practitioners. Others, however, chose quite the reverse approach: to utilize the opportunity created by the Dagmar mechanism to contract out new segments of primary care provision to the private sector. Moreover, this second group of counties chose to contract with the new, for-profit, corporate sector for these increased services, often in an explicit effort to create a fiscal and service quality comparison with the existing publicly operated health sector (Saltman, 1990). Swedish counties have the legal right to contract out service provision, and many have done so in the past in non-clinical health (ambulance, laundry, laboratory) and non-health areas (von Otter *et al.*, 1989). The advent of Dagmar-generated funds, however, provided the resources to initiate a much wider variety of service delivery experiments.

The Dagmar process, implemented by a Social Democratic government with centre (Agrarian) support with the objective of consolidating public sector planning and financial control, in practice was instrumental in developing a new and innovative private ambulatory sector, especially in counties governed by non-socialist majorities. As such, this reform became a key contributing factor to a new era of organizational variation that illustrates an emerging political pluralism at the county council level.

County experiments with private providers

Following upon the Dagmar Reform, a number of county councils began pilot projects with privately operated companies, seeking to explore potential financial efficiencies in private management or ownership of health delivery facilities. These projects typically involved the delivery of clinical services by an incorporated for-profit firm on a short-term contract basis – a form of privatization that differed considerably from the traditional pre-1970 Swedish private sector, which consisted predominantly of physicians in solo practice.

The new form of corporatization experiments first became

apparent in 1983 with the establishment in Stockholm of the City-Akuten ambulatory clinic. City-Akuten provides an interesting case study of how corporate-style privatization has developed within Sweden's publicly operated health system. Its clinic is located in the centre of Stockholm to provide care close to where large numbers of people work. The demand for its services has been very high, reflecting a growing 'individual want' to receive care quickly, without appointment and near to one's regular workplace. Similar services have been established in other large cities, though with less economic success.

Fees for City-Akuten's services have been paid (since 1985) by the county council out of its capitated Dagmar funds for ambulatory care. Patients pay only the same small fee that is required for an office visit at a public primary care centre. The physicians who staff City-Akuten are typically fully salaried to the public system, working in this private clinic during off-hours and vacation periods. This released time can run to four months a year, reflecting a county council decision in the late 1970s to compensate physicians with time off rather than with increased salaries.

Despite its formal status as a 'private' firm, then, the success of the Stockholm City-Akuten clinic directly reflects the fact that it serves predominantly public sector patients and operates almost entirely with public sector resources: it is staffed by public employees, utilizing public-sector-created off-duty time, and is paid with publicly collected and distributed funds. It is this dependent (proponents would argue symbiotic) relationship between public finance and private provision that demarcates most post-Dagmar private sector initiatives and gives recent Swedish experiments their unique character.

A different type of initiative has involved the direct contracting out of services to private providers. While there was some previous experience with private provision of auxiliary and support services, since 1985 there has been increasing experimentation with competitive bidding for core clinical services like primary health care and elective surgery. In both areas one can now find examples of for-profit, cooperative and established public providers participating in the competitive process.

With regard to primary health care, as of July 1990 about 50 per cent of the county councils were experimenting with at least one private provider model – a situation which reflects the rapid pace of change in policy direction. In Stockholm, experiences with private primary care have been mixed: one newly constructed health centre in a suburban area was contracted out to a single physician entrepreneur in 1988. However, an attempt by Stockholm County to put an existing health centre in a poorer neighbourhood out to bid succeeded in attracting only one submission, and that at a considerably higher capitation rate than present county expenditures. There was an instance in which the operators of a newly contracted-out health centre became bankrupt before opening. Other private initiatives are currently underway or are likely to be pursued despite the change in 1988 from a centre–right to a socialist-led county government.

Halland County in western Sweden also took early advantage of the primary care capitation system created by the 1985 Dagmar Reform to contract out one primary care centre – in the city of Halmstad – to a private physician group. Unlike the Stockholm experiment, the Halland contract was on a fee-for-service basis, with a reduction in per-unit payments after a certain volume per month. In an evaluation report, two consultants concluded that this private station had 'more than double as high productivity' as did three comparable publicly operated health centres, based upon statistics showing that the private centre saw more patients per hour (Stenberg and Åhgren, 1987). Partly on the basis of this controversial report, several counties opened negotiations to privatize health centres.

Corporately organized private provision of services in Sweden is not limited to ambulatory office visits: experiments in the private provision of inpatient hospital care are also underway. Örebro County, among others, sends public patients to the private Scandinavian Heart Centre in Göteborg, established in 1983 for coronary bypass surgery. In a similar pattern to the ambulatory model developed by City-Akuten, these cardiac operations are performed by off-duty surgeons salaried to the nearby Sahlgrenska University Hospital (Schildt, 1988). Stockholm County has begun to send patients waiting for elective surgery to the private sector. Since 1985, it has accepted bids from Sophiahemmet (a 150-bed privately owned hospital in Stockholm with a long tradition of private care) for full hip replacements and corneal lens implants. The county also negotiated contracts with several smaller entrepreneurial 'clinics' for hips and for lens implants. In 1990, 60 per cent of the counties were using external providers for elective surgery – a figure double that for 1989.

Stockholm County has also begun to contract out coronary bypass operations. In the spring of 1988, it purchased 50 operations from Sophiahemmet and – in a pattern now seen elsewhere in the Nordic region – 50 from the London-based for-profit multinational company American Medical International (AMI). The all-exclusive bid price from AMI, including round-trip airfare from Stockholm to London and two weeks in a hotel for an accompanying relative, was accepted as preferable to a rival bid from a newly formed 'weekend group' of cardiac surgeons at the Karolinska University Hospital, who sought to perform additional procedures on a for-profit basis in their publicly owned operating theatres during off-duty time (B. Könberg, private communication). This last model, of publicly employed physicians reconfiguring themselves on a for-profit part-time basis but in public facilities, is currently on trial in a variety of hospital settings elsewhere in Sweden.

The pre-eminent organization in Sweden's corporate health sector is Praktikertjänst AB, a privately owned for-profit company. Although founded in 1959 with the assistance of the Swedish Medical Association, in an effort to support private practitioners after the 1955 reform, Praktikertjänst blossomed in the 1980s into the major private provider of ambulatory health services in Sweden. In terms of patient volume, Praktikertjänst provides approximately half of the three million private ambulatory care visits in Sweden, or about 5 per cent of all primary care visits nationally (SCB, 1988). It also delivers more than one-third of all dental care in Sweden, through some 2200 dental offices (50 per cent of the private dental offices in Sweden). In terms of financial performance, Praktikertjänst more than doubled its annual revenues between 1980 and 1987 (Praktikertjänst AB, 1980, 1987). This growth included income from a variety of satellite companies, including its own internal bank.

Praktikertjänst is structured as a closely held corporation, with stock ownership restricted to health professionals who bring their private practice into the company. In spring 1988, the company had some 935 stockholders. Health professionals who leave the company for any reason are required to sell their shares back to the company at an annually determined par value. Moreover, the company does not pay out dividends. Rather, it invests annual 'profit' from each individual provider office (i.e. income after office expenses and corporate management fees) in a corporately held

reserve fund which, upon the owning health professional's retirement, will be paid out as a private pension. Since this reserve fund
accumulates interest that is untaxed, it enables the member
physician to transfer a substantial portion of his or her office's
annual operating profit directly into retirement income. Pra-
tikertjänst thus views itself as a type of 'provider cooperative', not
only in its internal organization but also in its restriction of stock
ownership to member health professionals.

Overall, this newly corporatized private sector has remained
marginal (Rosenthal, 1986, 1990). There has been, however, clear
growth in the number of elective surgical procedures which have
been contracted out to private providers, a trend which recent
experience in the United Kingdom has demonstrated can present
serious planning as well as political complications for a publicly
operated health system (Nicholl *et al.*, 1984). In Stockholm County
public costs for private ambulatory visits have increased by 68 per
cent in three years (*Dagens Nyheter*, 3 August 1989).

A key question concerns the fate of public needs in this
profit-making planned market model. The example of City-Akuten
is frequently cited by proponents of private sector contracting to
prove that private providers can be made to satisfy public objectives
through carefully designed reimbursement controls. Similarly, the
closely held 'producer' character of Praktikertjänst, largely in-
sulated from external capital market pressures, could be viewed as
further confirmation that a resurgent private delivery sector need
not generate the uncontrolled corporatization in Sweden that
occurred during the 1980s in the United States (Whiteis and
Salmon, 1987). This type of evidence, however, cannot satisfac-
torily resolve the broader theoretical questions involved in the
private provision of public sector human services (Saltman and von
Otter, 1987), issues with which the Swedish counties have yet to
grapple.

One consequence of current experiments with private providers
has been their impact on the willingness of public sector providers to
adopt more flexible patterns of organization. County-level administrators and politicians have become more receptive to 'intre-
preneurs' within the public system who have come forward with
innovative ideas about institutional structures and working
patterns. This 'spill-over effect' has also encouraged public sector
unions and Federation of County Council officials to entertain once
unacceptable proposals to develop more flexible forms of health

service delivery in the public sector. We explore this process in some detail in the next section.

County experiments with public providers

Concurrent with post-Dagmar experiments to purchase contracted services from private providers, a number of Swedish counties have also begun to explore new planning and management techniques within existing public service provision. Although these efforts are still in the developmental phase, a number of counties have begun to introduce planned market elements within one or more sub-sectors of the public health care system. If these initiatives take root they could well transform the Swedish health system from one of the most uniform to among the most pluralist publicly operated systems in Europe.

The counties' initial agenda began with increasing interest in budgetary systems which could parlay patient choice into more cost-effective service delivery, and enhance options for patient choice within primary and hospital level services. Allowing patients some degree of latitude over where and from whom they receive their health care is now the rule within the Swedish county councils. The effective extent of patient choice, however, varies considerably between different county councils, between different levels of services (hospital, primary and social services) and between particular activities within each service level. As a result there is now an increasing number of opportunities for Swedish citizens to influence the conditions under which they receive care. Although certain opportunities are recent in nature, others which officially have been possible for some time are now being made more generally available.

While the existence of official opportunities need not necessarily be congruent with real opportunities to exercise choice of provider or, more commonly, of site of care, there is now increasing political pressure to ensure that patient choice is not obstructed by intra-county political or organizational resistance. In what represented an important shift of political strategy within the national Social Democratic party, the Minister of Health supported patient choice at every level of service delivery. Speaking in a parliamentary debate in spring 1988, the Minister made the national government's position, as well as the logic behind it, quite explicit: 'People should be able to visit the doctor, the health centre, or the hospital they wish, also across county lines. Attempts with such choice have been shown to reduce the demand for private alternatives' (*Landstingsvärlden*, August 1988, p. 33). The Federation of County Councils issued a declaration in 1989 to the same effect (Landstingsförbundet, 1989), which resulted in official implementation of the principle of patient choice within all counties from January 1991. A number of counties have also widened patient choice across county lines, particularly in the southern and western parts of the country (*Landstingsvärlden*, 24 January 1991, pp. 14–15).

The results from two studies, in May 1988 (von Otter *et al.*, 1989) and spring 1990, point up an uneven picture regarding the extent to which patient choice has been exercised within the Swedish health system. In the primary care sector, patients appear to have had considerably more ability to choose the particular physician from whom they receive care than to choose the actual site of care. Before the new arrangements in January 1991, Swedish patients had considerably greater formal than actual opportunities to select their provider, with substantially fewer options to change health centres either within or between counties. One exception had been a legal agreement among five adjacent counties in western Sweden which allowed patients to designate a primary care centre in any one of the participating counties (Västsvenska Planeringsnämnden, 1984). This agreement was necessitated by the complicated living and commuting patterns in the greater Gothenburg region.

With regard to outpatient (polyclinic) care, patients had considerably less official right to choose than in inpatient hospital areas. For scheduled inpatient care, patients were more likely to have some influence over site and provider, but the figures for out-of-county care may have reflected region-level university hospital treatment more than care at equivalent county-level general hospitals.

Before 1991, therefore, the overall impression was of a health system in which patient choice over provider and site, while certainly not extensive, was increasingly accepted in a variety of service activities. While this represented a considerable shift from prior practice within the Swedish publicly operated health system, changes underway in the 1990s have led to the institutionalization of patient choice as a standard aspect of Sweden's publicly operated system.

The picture with regard to new budgeting arrangements capable of transforming patient choice experiments into a more explicit planned market approach is less well developed, although a number of counties are working on new systems. In the primary care as well as outpatient and inpatient hospital sectors, and with regard to personal provider remuneration as well as delivery unit budgets, there are as yet few meaningful links between performance and productivity on the one hand and level of budget on the other. A similar lack of connection exists with regard to personnel salaries, although in all but three counties physicians and physician teams are now able to earn a performance-tied bonus. Several counties also attempt to adjust delivery unit budgets to reflect patient load and efficiency levels, but at present these adjustments tend to be quite limited (marginal operating costs only) and often are 'rescue measures' utilized at the end of the budget year. Taken together, these observations suggest the difficulty in changing vestigial planning and budgeting mechanisms that had little effective incentive for improved performance.

One perspective on current public sector experiments can be seen in ongoing efforts to restructure service provision in Stockholm County. While other county councils – including Malmöhus, Halland, Bohuslän and Östergötland – are becoming active in this area, the process of change to a new choice-driven public competition market model can be seen clearly in several experiments in Stockholm.

The Stockholm County initiatives on primary care allow individuals to select a regular health centre wherever they prefer in the county (*Dagens Nyheter*, 6 March 1989). In an 'experiment within an experiment', one central Stockholm primary care district has been reorganized into 25 general practitioner-led teams which provide curative and preventive services, partly on a walk-in basis (Rydén and Sjönell, 1989; Öhrming, 1990). With regard to inpatient hospital care, an initial experiment in the maternity sector began in January 1988, in which expectant mothers select in which of the county maternity units they would like to deliver. In the first half of 1990, 19 per cent of expectant mothers requested to be transferred (Karolinska Hospital, 1990). Of these, 25 per cent of those who had previously 'belonged' to one smaller hospital located on the western edge of the county chose to deliver elsewhere. This smaller hospital (Södertälje) as a consequence developed a substantial revenue shortfall (Karolinska Hospital, 1990). Another hospital, which previously offered only a highly medicalized delivery mode, rapidly remodelled some delivery rooms and introduced more natural delivery methods as an option where desired.

Viewed overall, this experiment succeeded in enabling patients to choose the facility at which they would receive care, based on location, reputation and general information about the practice style in each facility. Several maternity units found it to be in their own best interest to adopt a more interactive delivery approach. Inasmuch as operating revenues for all seven Stockholm maternity units became linked to performance, issues of internal efficiency and responsiveness to patients became an important element in how maternity units were managed.

This exercise of patient choice did not substantially change patient numbers in five of the seven facilities, but one highly respected facility increased numbers (Karolinska Hospital). The hospital that lost patient custom found itself under close scrutiny from central county administrators, and efforts were initiated to redress the loss of patient revenue. In order to remain open, this maternity clinic began to perform diagnostic tests on patients referred from another hospital with long queues for these procedures. When one delivery ward ultimately had to be closed, the decision was seen to be managerially necessary rather than a politically imposed process. The success of this experiment in turn has led to the development of the 'Stockholm model', which, if implemented as scheduled in 1991, will combine expanded patient choice of hospital site and provider with primary care based controls over hospital reimbursement. This new arrangement will be roughly similar in structure to the 'Dalarna model' in Kopparberg County (discussed below), but in Stockholm it appears that most if not all providers participating in the new planned market will be publicly operated and the administrative costs of contracts with hospital clinics will be minimized (*Landstingsvärlden*, 24 January 1991, pp. 11–12).

Both primary and hospital sector experiments in Stockholm County reflect a long-running administrative initiative to decentralize budgetary responsibility to each delivery unit, or *basenhet*, within provider institutions. These budgeting initiatives have now been directly linked to patient decisions regarding choice of services. In the primary and maternity services experiments, patient decisions to seek care have been followed by an additional budgetary payment to the provider institution, calculated as the additional marginal cost incurred. For primary care, the additional amount has been paid on a capitated annual patients basis, with the sum doubled for patients over age 65 (J.-E. Speck, personal communication). There is, however, no change in compensation for the staff at the provider institution as an incentive to serve additional patients. Further, there are no contemporaneous changes in budgetary allocation to provider institutions that lose patient volume. The current experiment thus involves only a positive or 'adaptive planning' form of budgetary linkage to patient-related performance. In Stockholm County, moreover, questions of patient choice and budgetary linkages have yet to involve payment for patient-selected services across county lines.

Another radical planned market reform is underway in Kopparberg County in the Dalarna region of central Sweden. As described in the proposal document (SIAR, 1990), this 'Dalamodel' is intended to achieve cost-effectiveness while at the same time strengthening the role of primary health services. This reform is scheduled to be fully introduced in January 1993.

The central mechanism of the Dalamodel is the administrative separation of primary health care from hospital care, through the creation of 15 primary health boards (composed of county politicians) designed to have the same borders as Kopparberg County's component municipalities. Each primary health care board will operate the primary health centre in its district, and purchase hospital services for district inhabitants. Since the boards will control both primary care and hospital budgets for district residents, the expectation is that the primary health centres attached to these new boards will be encouraged to reduce unnecessary referrals to hospital (in order to keep a portion of the hospital budget) and to monitor the necessity of specialist services provided to referred patients. Moreover, the model introduces a contract relationship designed to put pressure on hospital clinics to reduce their operating costs as a means to retain primary care centre referrals. In an innovative approach, 'population responsibility' (*befolkningsansvar*) will now rest with the local district boards, while hospital clinics and primary health centres will have a more limited 'results responsibility' (*resultatansvar*) linked directly to productivity.

Two additional elements of the Dalamodel involve the introduction of patient choice and performance incentives. Individuals will be assigned annually to a primary health centre according to their residential district (for the purpose of developing the annual budget), but they will be able to enrol as regular patients at any other health centre, with the cost carried by their 'home' health centre. In order to make private ambulatory visits, individuals will be required to pay a small supplemental charge out-of-pocket, but most of the cost will also be defrayed from the 'home' health centre's budget. Finally, with regard to inpatient hospital services, the Kopparberg proposal will officially allow patients to choose among existing in-county institutions, but is unclear about the ability of patients to elect out-of-county or private hospital clinics.

The Dalamodel includes direct financial incentives to health care personnel for improved performance, in the form of bonus payments. The proposal's emphasis upon new marginal incentives to fixed salaries reflects the pragmatic realities of existing national labour union contracts as well as sitting politicians' electoral sensitivities.

Three observations can be made about the Dalamodel as proposed. First, the structural emphasis upon the 'home' health centre may generate both positive and negative outcomes when the model is introduced. Positively, the clearly visible record of each health centre's overall performance, as assessed by patient decisions to obtain care at alternative sites, will harness a powerful non-financial incentive – professional prestige – to improve health centre ratings. Negatively, the notion of 'home' health centres can create pressure from health professionals for patients to forgo their formal right to visit another health centre. 'Home' health centre personnel may imply that it would be preferable not to seek care elsewhere, on grounds that such shifts would deprive them of an overview of the health needs of the entire local population.

A second point concerns the potential conflict that may emerge between patient preference of hospital clinic, on the one hand, and established contracts between that patient's local health board and a particular hospital clinic, on the other. Whether patient choice, based primarily on quality, rather than the local board contract, based primarily on price, will prevail is not clear.

A third comment concerns the administrative expense of requiring local boards to negotiate contracts for each category of patient treatment and then to monitor the outcome. If this requirement is implemented, there might need to be substantially increased administrative resources at each local board and hospital clinic, diverting considerable funding from clinical use. Further, the ability and motivation of physicians to negotiate contracts that adquately define quality can vary greatly depending upon the type of services in question (Schlesinger *et al.*, 1987).

CONCLUSION

The Swedish health system is in the midst of substantial structural and organizational transition. The Höjer-based policy period, with its emphasis upon an allocative planning system and prioritization of publicly produced primary health care, appears to be approaching its end. Current county council experiments with different planned market approaches, in particular with new provider models like those in Stockholm and Kopparberg, as well as structural changes in the financial system involving sickness pay and workers' compensation, suggest that the future shape of the delivery system has yet to be determined. This organizational openness is reinforced by current debate about the system's structural configuration, including the role of county (regional) *vis-à-vis* both national and municipal governments and the proper national–local balance for policy and administrative issues.

This period of experimentation has been triggered by the 1983 Health Act and the Dagmar Reform which, by channelling national funding for ambulatory physician care through independent county councils, created a powerful financial incentive for planned market experimentation. In an environment characterized by conflicting pressures of economy, demography, technology and social preference, the Dagmar funding mechanism became an ideal first step in the process of health sector re-design. However, the Dagmar Reform will inevitably require further reform measures if the current set of contradictory financial incentives is to be rationalized.

Dagmar did accomplish its central administrative objective, which was to cap ambulatory care budgets. If only for fiscal reasons, neither non-socialist nor socialist-led counties are interested in surrendering their new Dagmar-generated authority. Concurrently, however, the broader political goal of Dagmar, which was to strengthen public health care planning and the national primary care strategy, is now in the hands of the 26 different county governments. It may well be that, in the contrast between Dagmar's administrative and political outcomes, one can see the high-water mark of the movement towards a fully public delivery system in Sweden. In this assessment, the Dagmar process facilitated the return of private practitioners and private sector beds to the Swedish health system in the mid-1980s.

The future shape of the health sector in Sweden, and the precise characteristics of a new dominant model, are increasingly visible in current planned market projects. Different approaches, in terms of the market-based incentive harnessed, the agent of change selected and the particular public/private mix, are under development and, increasingly, in use. Current experiments are partial and tentative, however, often lacking clear links to the major salary and budget determination processes that drive decisions inside the county organizations. None the less, an overwhelming majority of counties have now accepted the usefulness of introducing at least some planned market elements into their delivery patterns. As existing experiments mature into more comprehensive planned market frameworks, the criteria for evaluation of and selection among differing alternatives may become more apparent to national, county and municipal level officials.

In the Swedish instance, there are no signs that the present process of experimentation will trigger a dramatic shift to a USA-style for-profit or insurance-based delivery system. The key issues for health sector reform in Sweden parallel those for the other human service sectors, and it appears that a set of common answers is emerging across political party lines (Leijon and Eklund, 1989; Framtidsgruppen, 1989). For all the breadth of Dagmar-induced experimentation, the publicly accountable, tax-based character of the health system has not been seriously questioned. There remain, however, important questions about the long-term incremental consequences of a growing private sector presence. Quick to recognize and exploit a vacuum, private providers have sought to develop their role rapidly and to restore their legitimacy within the Swedish health system. They have accomplished this latter goal to the degree that the health sector officials accept some private sector participation as appropriate. Statements by national officials about the importance of a private comparison and the usefulness of a 'complementary' private sector give the private sector confidence about its future. As Swedish initiatives with planned markets continue to evolve, however, it seems increasingly unlikely that the private sector's role will grow beyond serving as a helpful prod to a revitalized public system.

5

PLANNING AND MARKETS IN FINLAND

THE POLICY CONTEXT

The Finnish health care system emerged in the 1980s as an internationally acknowledged prototype for a publicly planned delivery system. Following upon its successful effort to build up primary care and preventive services through a system of publicly funded, publicly operated health centres, Finland was selected by the World Health Organization as a model country in 1982, and key elements subsequently developed for the Health for All strategy in WHO's European region bore a strong resemblance to the Finnish approach (WHO, 1984).

This emphasis upon the publicly planned and operated characteristics of the Finnish model has tended to underemphasize a number of lateral and contradictory pressures that were built into the Finnish system, and that continued to affect the process of planning, financing and delivering necessary services. With regard to planning, the powerful subsidy-tied planning process established at the national level by the 1972 Primary Care Act created considerable tension with municipal governments, who officially owned, and were obligated by legislation to provide approximately 50 per cent funding for, both primary care and hospital facilities. As one ministry official noted in a 1986 interview, 'In theory, we haven't taken away the autonomy of the commune, but in practice we have' (Saltman, 1988a).

With regard to financing, the national–municipal tax-based system for primary health centres and hospitals is only one of two separately funded, separately administered, but publicly accountable health care revenue streams. The Social Insurance Institution, established in 1964 and funded via mandatory payroll taxes, provides per-visit subsidies for private ambulatory visits (60 per cent of the officially scheduled but arbitrarily low tariff), private inpatient treatment (a fixed amount per procedure, perhaps 10–25 per cent of 1990 costs) and occupational health services – including primary care visits to company physicians – provided by both private and public employers (55 per cent of actual operating costs). A further public financing of private and occupational health expenditures is provided through the national tax system, which allows direct deductions from taxable income for private individuals (up to 2000 Finnmarks per year) and corporations.

Private health insurance, no doubt reflecting the availability of social insurance subsidies, is not particularly well developed in Finland. Beyond a small number of well-off urban inhabitants, most private policies are taken out by parents for their children, an apparently common middle-class practice to guarantee immediate access to acute ambulatory or elective inpatient care.

Finally, with regard to service delivery, and directly reflecting available financing mechanisms, Finland continues to have a substantial private primary care and a small but rapidly growing private hospital sector. There are private polyclinics in the bigger cities, and a substantial number of publicly employed health centre physicians maintain private practices in the evenings. Although private hospitals had been largely limited to one 150-bed institution – Mehiläinen – and three smaller facilities in Helsinki, the last years of the 1980s saw a profileration of new small surgical hospitals, typically founded by specialist physicians in university-hospital cities. Publicly operated hospitals also maintain a few private beds in each clinic, for which no additional charges are made but to which senior physicians' private patients can be admitted (thereby jumping the queue). A parallel development has been a growing number of patients travelling abroad under various public and private payment arrangements for elective procedures like coronary by-pass surgery.

Part of the overall success of Finland's publicly planned and operated health system during the 1970s and early 1980s was that public and private policy cross-pressures did not seriously affect the continued development of the public system. The public sector was in an expansionary mode, additional national and local revenues were available for discretionary services like health care, and popular cultural concerns were focused on issues of equity and social justice. Indeed, until the late 1980s, the publicly operated system was seen to be in the ascendant and privately delivered health services seemed increasingly vestigial and unimportant.

In 1989 and 1990 the health policy process in Finland changed direction. The external pressures described in Chapter 1 which confront other publicly operated systems – constraints of demography, technology and economy – combined with the mixed structure of the Finnish health system to create a volatile and seemingly unanticipated set of reversals in policy orientation. The social insurance and private sector suddenly bulked more prominently in future delivery plans, while the publicly operated system increasingly appeared distracted and directionless. The new situation was symbolized by the unwillingness of a growing number of graduating medical students to take up posts in the publicly operated health centres. Their absence, in combination with a sizeable number of resignations by appointed physicians in the primary health centres, led to a growing number of badly understaffed health centres. In summer 1990, some disillusioned physicians in Helsinki contended that fully one-third of all health centre physicians had resigned over the previous five-year period. A May 1990 report from the National Board of Health indicated 700 official vacancies for general practitioners, and chief physicians in a number of health centres reported privately that it had become difficult to hire temporary replacement physicians to help out during the summer vacation period. As a consequence, there was growing concern about the long-term viability of the publicly operated primary care system.

To be sure, the publicly operated system remains the dominant service delivery structure in Finland, and few seriously question the continued existence of at least an overwhelmingly public hospital system. In its official statements, the national government supports continued development of the publicly operated system, and it has strengthened its commitment to pursue the WHO Health for All strategy in Finland (Finnish Ministry of Social Affairs and Health, 1987). There are also several policy initiatives underway that seek to revitalize the public primary care system, and that have shown a degree of success in initial trials. There is, finally, the intangible but essential role of public opinion and the overall spirit of the times, and thus a continuing possibility of reform in the publicly operated system.

RECENT STRUCTURAL INNOVATIONS

The discussion below concentrates on three central elements of the present structural problem in Finland. The first is a process of administrative consolidation within the public sector which is underway at the national, hospital district and municipal levels. The second is the development of new organizational patterns for physicians inside the public health centres, in an effort to rethink the negative inertial biases of a rigidly bureaucratic primary care system. The third, and clearly the most important, is the accelerating devolution of the national health planning process to the municipal level. These three structural changes together illustrate the conflicting policy pressures that have now combined to produce proposals for a fundamental restructuring of the Finnish health system.

Administrative Consolidation

Public agencies in the Finnish health sector have been engaged in a notably broad process of administrative consolidation since the mid-1980s. While the central purpose of this process initially reflected the primary care orientation of the national government's Health for All strategy, and the consequent interest in integrating social services into the health planning mechanism, subsequent changes suggest that governmental efforts to obtain more direct political control over health-related decision-making have become an equal if not more important objective.

At the national level, the consolidation of social services into health planning took effect in January 1985. While this provided additional national subsidies for health-related social and home care, it also injected the National Board of Health (which drew up the national plan) and the Ministry of Social Affairs and Health (which approved it) directly into the municipalities' administration of all social services. Among other intrusions, it meant that municipalities lost practical control over their ability to invest available local funds as well as matched national subsidies into child or old-age housing rather than health-related home care services, since operating and capital spending decisions for the latter (and thus municipal expenditures for home-care) were stipulated in the national plan (Saltman, 1988a). This consolidation of national planning control helped to trigger a municipal reaction against the entire national planning process in spring 1987 (see below).

This combined national plan led to two further administrative changes, both of which were underway in 1990, one at national and the other at local level. The first was the integration of the National Board of Health with the National Board of Social Welfare. Although this consolidation could be viewed as a logical administrative step once health and social service planning had been consolidated, the decision can be interpreted as part of a longer-term effort by the ministry to reduce the policy independence and, in practice, the role of the senior medical professionals who staffed the National Board of Health. Certainly, the decision to remove responsibility for the national planning process to the ministry, and to halve the number of total positions to 200, suggests a diminished role for the new combined board in policy formulation. Viewed historically, the Finnish decision more or less parallels the administrative arrangement established in Sweden in 1969, with the creation of the joint National Board of Health and Welfare (known in Swedish as Socialstyrelsen or, literally 'social steering agency'). Whether the consolidated Finnish board will be able to duplicate the recent success of its Swedish counterpart in carving out a major role for itself in monitoring and evaluating health services delivery remains to be seen.

The second consolidation process is at the municipal level, where efforts to combine local political boards responsible for supervising health and social services have gained momentum. Of the approximately 100 municipalities that have their own health boards (municipalities in primary health care federations participate in the federation council instead), 24 have combined their social and health boards; 21 took this step in 1989. Much like the efforts taken at the national level, this consolidation seeks to increase the capacity of public officials to monitor the still largely independent planning and operating behaviour of the social service and health sectors.

Structural change at the third, intermediate, level has focused on the administrative arrangements by which the municipalities own and operate Finland's hospitals. Although no action has thus far been taken on proposals to reform the role of the provincial governments (Saltman, 1988a), which serve as the regional administrative arm of the national government and are staffed by appointed civil servants, the configuration of hospital federations was changed as of January 1991. From a myriad of separate municipal federations, one for each free-standing tertiary (central), secondary (district), mental and (vestigial) tuberculosis facility, each with its own separate administrative board and budget, there are now 22 specialist hospital districts which contain all referral institutions within their respective boundaries.

These districts are structured as municipal federations, but they have relatively strong central administrations that are empowered to refer patients to whichever of Finland's five university hospitals the district administration prefers. Beyond this contract role for university hospital patients, these district administrators may also be able to contract out their own central hospital patients to other (public) specialist hospital districts or to private sector institutions. Even without the authority to contract out central hospital patients (there is still some dispute inside Finland about this), these specialist hospital districts apparently will in certain respects have a role similar to district health authorities in the UK under the 1990 NHS and Community Care Act, in that they will be able to rationalize individual institutions as well as to contract out at least some groups of patients.

While these specialist hospital districts were originally intended to simplify and rationalize the Finnish hospital sector's administrative structure, this new arrangement has been transformed by the present volatile context into an important policy event. There are concerns among defenders of Finland's primary health oriented strategy that these new hospital districts will marshal their physicians' prestige and their large revenue base to overwhelm the primary health centres. It is also unclear whether this reform will enhance municipal ability to control (if not manage) the specialist institutions that local governments technically own and fund, which officially was a related goal of the reform, or whether the new consolidated structure will only exacerbate the traditional inability of local politicians to penetrate the tight self-governing cocoon created by physician-led hospital administrations (Saltman, 1988a). Finally, depending on whether the specialist hospital districts will generate a contract-based market for university and – under some interpretations of the new law – central hospital patients, there are concerns about whether this administrative reform may in fact create a UK-style mixed market in Finland.

These structural consolidations (with the exception of possible contracting abilities of the specialist hospital districts) were conceived primarily as efforts to shake up existing administrative components and to reassemble them in a more integrated and efficient command-and-control manner. There have been two further charges in the administrative structure of the Finnish system, which have helped create the context within which this process of administrative consolidation has occurred. We review each of these aspects in turn.

Personal Doctor Programme

The national planning apparatus in Finland has invested considerable effort in a series of projects to improve the quality of health services by reforming existing physician payment systems. The linchpin of efforts regarding general practitioners was a long-running demonstration project called the Personal Doctor Programme (Vohlonen *et al.*, 1989). The demonstration sought to test three different models of ways to reorganize the delivery of primary care into a list-based system, in which individuals (the Finnish programme refers to them as 'citizens') enrol with a specific general practitioner from whom they receive care. Two of these models were tested in publicly operated health centres, while one was utilized by private sector general practitioners. Model 1 created a list-based system inside the selected health centres but without altering the standard 100 per cent salary basis of physician compensation. Model 2 linked a list-based system to a tripartite physician reimbursement system, in which compensation for general practitioners comprised: (a) a basic allowance for education and experience (20 per cent); (b) a capitation allowance reflecting the size and the age and sex adjusted characteristics of each physician's list (60 per cent); (c) a coverage allowance determined by the percentage of a physician's total list seen at least once during the payment period (20 per cent). Model 3, which was designed for private sector general practitioners, utilized a list-based compensation system parallel to that tested in the public system in model 2, with an additional supplement to reimburse the private physicians' auxiliary medical staff. To insure the comparability of results, arrangements were also made so that patients utilizing private sector physicians did not have to make co-payments for physician visits.

This Personal Doctor Programme was intended to achieve an interconnected set of policy objectives. First and foremost, the programme sought to improve the continuity of care received by patients in the publicly operated system. While continuity was particularly important to patients with chronic conditions (who visit their physician regularly) and to the elderly, planners believed that greater continuity would improve the general quality of primary care received, and hence overall patient satisfaction with the delivery system. Further, improved patient continuity generated by a list-based system was perceived to be an important factor in physician satisfaction, allowing general practitioners to 'build a practice' inside a health centre much like that of private physicians, with a concomitant sense of responsibility and accomplishment. Increased physician satisfaction was particularly important to combat the problem of psychological exhaustion or 'burn-out', which had become increasingly cited as a consequence of the prior 'assembly-line' approach to patient care (Piri and Vohlonen, 1987). Finally, and as important as the preceding reasons, the linkage of physician compensation to performance in terms of size of list and population coverage (parts (b) and (c) of the model 2 programme) was expected to increase internal efficiency inside publicly operated health centres.

This combination of expected benefits – improved continuity and quality of care, greater patient and physician satisfaction, and enhanced operating efficiency – suggests that the Personal Doctor Programme ought to have made a major contribution to the Finnish primary care system. This contribution was confirmed by an evaluation of the first phase (1985–7) of the programme, which indicated that: (a) list-based systems were superior on each assessed index to their non-list control counterparts; (b) public health centre physicians with performance-related compensation (model 2) generated the greatest overall value for funds expended (Vohlonen *et al.*, 1989); and (c) health centre physicians uniformly preferred the model 2 arrangement not so much because it raised their overall compensation (by approximately 10 per cent after taxes), but because it liberated them from the rigid hourly productivity norms which had previously been utilized (M. Liukko, personal communication).

Although the Personal Doctor Programme went through a second phase demonstration (1987–90), it was supplanted in 1990 by a national government programme called the Small Area Based Population Responsibility Programme (SABPRP). In this reconfigured programme, primary health and primary medical activities are included, although there is no new performance-related compensation system for nurses and other members of primary care teams. Key features of a revised ambulatory physician's contract include a modified version of the tripartite compensation model, with the capitation allowance being modified to incorporate only those patients who make two or more GP visits per year. The third reimbursement segment has now become a two part fee-for-service mechanism for (a) patients who visit only once in a year, and (b) a small number of specified procedures (for example, examining a suspected drunk driver at police request). This new programme was in place in ten experimental sites in December 1989 (S. Aro, personal communication).

The new GP contract will place the third of all citizens who are responsible for 80–90 per cent of ambulatory physician visits in the capitation-based system. Conversely, the increment for specific procedures is anticipated to affect approximately 5 per cent of total physician compensation. There will be only one physician compensation model for public health centre and private general practitioners alike, modified to include in its third segment an element of direct fee-for-service reimbursement.

One indication of the shift in Finnish health policy at the end of the 1980s can be seen in the changed structure and expectations from the original Personal Doctor Programme to those now held for the replacement SABPRP. When it was initially conceived in 1985, the Personal Doctor Programme was viewed by national planning officials as a logical next step in achieving the objectives of Finland's primary health care policy. The mechanism of paying personal doctors was seen as secondary to the programme's central objective of generating higher levels of continuity of care and patient and provider satisfaction. Further, an unstated political objective of the programme was to make public health centres so efficient and well-respected that they would limit the future growth of the private ambulatory sector.

With the shift in the health policy context in 1989 and 1990, efforts to reform physician workloads and reimbursement acquired not only a new configuration but also a more central policy brief. Faced with growing dissatisfaction with the publicly operated primary health centres, an inability to recruit sufficient numbers of primary care physicians, and substantial cost-generated pressures to improve the health system's efficiency and productivity, the SABPRP is now described by some primary care advocates as a critical element for the survival of the publicly operated health centre system. A municipal health official in one city in central Finland, for example, worried that the local health centre system might not survive until the new arrangement could be put in place.

At the same time that this new set of expectations emerged, key tenets of the original Personal Doctor Programme were undercut in the replacement programme by proponents of a traditional needs-based planning approach. In response to fears that the original Personal Doctor Programme's incentive structure would fragment the 'population responsibility' that planners view as essential to a community-oriented preventive approach, the SABPRP recreates core elements of the traditional command-and-control planning approach within smaller health centre sub-districts. In particular, citizens are once again more or less tied by their place of residence to a provider 'team' made up of a physician, nurses and social service personnel, with only minimal choice among the available sub-district providers. While survey data suggests only 5 per cent would like to change their assigned physicians, patients in these experimental areas obtain 40–60 per cent of their ambulatory physician care from private physicians and/or outpatient clinics (S. Aro, personal communication).

In a number of municipalities disputes have led officials to ignore the incentive payment element in the programme, and to continue to pay all members of the primary care team a fixed salary unrelated to any measure of patient volume or productivity. Nor will these local primary care teams have a decentralized budget, quite unlike the Swedish primary care experiments. In effect, although the SABPRP has reinforced the health system's focus upon the principles of population-based preventive care, it has undercut the patient-choice-tied-to-provider-incentive component of the original Personal Doctor approach. Whether this renewed command-and-control administrative model will suffice to restore momentum to the Finnish public primary care system remains to be seen.

Devolution of the national plan

A crucial element in establishing the preconditions for the recent shift in the health policy balance has been concerted efforts by Finnish municipalities to loosen the national government's health planning grip. In Finland as elsewhere, this tension between central and local government is long-standing, and is not limited exclusively to the health sector. None the less, tight national controls over new health sector resources provoked increasingly strong resistance from both municipalities and their local health institutions.

The first (and continuing) step in defiance of the national planning process has involved efforts by wealthier municipalities to build new capital facilities 'off-budget'. Under the national plan, all official capital expenditures had to be approved by either the provincial (over 4 million Finnmarks) or the national (11 million later increased to 14 million Finnmarks) government. Capital was tightly rationed, and the common understanding was that 'it took ten years to build' in the Finnish health system (Saltman, 1988a). By the mid-1980s some municipalities began to evade this capital control process entirely by setting up publicly owned companies, which borrowed funds from the municipality or banks, built the desired facility and then leased it back to the health centre or hospital. One small Finnish city utilized this arrangement to build, among other facilities, a new health centre building (45 million Finnmarks), a shared central laundry and a hospital pharmacy (20 million Finnmarks).

A second, more explicit step in the devolution of the national plan occurred in spring 1987. Unable or unwilling to pay for increased growth as mandated by the national plan, the municipalities revolted. Instead of accepting the 1988 plan as proposed, the municipalities sent the plan back to the National Board of Health to be redrafted. Among municipal demands was an insistence that the rigid delineation of new posts – one of the Finnish planning process's two core mechanisms (Saltman, 1988a) – be 'melted' to allow the municipalities leeway to assign allotted posts where they felt was most appropriate. While this change did not affect the strict budgetary segregation between hospital, primary care and social service sub-sectors (each of which receives its budget from a different administrative entity in a majority of Finnish municipalities), the new 'softer' boundaries allowed a primary care federation, for example, to hire a new nurse instead of requiring the municipality to add a home care worker to its social service. As it turned out, this revised planning process, adopted in January 1990, had only two personnel categories: one for physicians (ostensibly to ration the shortage), the second for 'other health personnel'.

A third set of events which undercut the national plan reflects various extra-system efforts to reduce queues for elective surgery, particularly for coronary by-pass procedures. Central hospitals

have allowed fully salaried surgeons to establish 'private' companies to work on nights and weekends, and negotiated arrangements to use public funds to send patients to a private hospital in
Helsinki (Mehiläinen) as well as abroad to London and (at the
urging of the National Board of Health) to Pamplona in Spain and
Talinn in Estonia. Although all these efforts were 'approved' by the
national government, they were ironically seen in some quarters as
confirmation of the rigidities of the national planning process
(which had sought to ration resources for elective inpatient care in
pursuit of revenues to develop primary care) and the consequent
inadequacies of the publicly operated hospitals. Most importantly,
they added fuel to the private health sector fire, which in 1989 and
1990 erupted into a number of new private surgical hospitals (all of
which, it should be mentioned, have been approved by the
provincial and therefore the national government). The most
salient example is the January 1991 opening of a 16-bed coronary
heart surgery hospital in Kuopio, constructed with 24 million
borrowed Finnmarks, and with expectations of long-term contracts
from several hospital districts in central Finland.

Taken together, these three structural developments – administrative consolidation, the Personal Doctor Programme and the
devolution of the national plan – represent a substantial shift in the
organizational configuration of the Finnish health system. It is
testimony to the pressures which are now driving the process of
change in Finland's publicly operated health system that these
reforms are likely to be only the beginning of a prolonged period of
health system reconfiguration. As the following discussion suggests,
the three recent structural reforms may well serve only to set the
stage for the next, perhaps main, set of events.

FUTURE ISSUES

The present health policy debate in Finland directly reflects the
changing balance between the former, centrally planned approach
and a mixed public and private, decentralized, market-influenced
organizational arrangement. Whether this shifting focus of power
reflects the triumph as well as the apparent demise of Finland's
central planning process is, however, unclear. It could be argued
that, having developed a well-articulated, publicly operated health
system over nearly a 20-year period, the national plan has served its

intended purpose and should now surrender control to the system's rightful owners, the municipalities (Saltman, 1988a). Others, particularly national officials concerned about the willingness and ability of many local governments to sustain the Finnish system's emphasis upon primary, preventive and population based health as against narrowly curative medical care, are less sanguine about the end of national planning. Certainly, the ongoing shift suggests that the political hegemony of policy-makers who came into the Finnish national government in the early 1970s – what might be termed the 'planning generation' – may well be ending.

It is important to emphasize that the present policy debate reflects a continued strong public presence in the health sector. Moreover, most of the proposed changes involve consolidation of financing and administrative responsibility in the hands of the municipalities. In this key respect, the shifting balance of decision-making authority in Finland appears to be strengthening local public control and accountability if not the existing publicly operated delivery system. The implications of this new emphasis can be seen in two major issues under debate during 1990 – the so-called Hiltunen Plan to create a block-grant financing system, and a Ministry of Social Affairs and Health proposal to create a local planning and management office within each municipality – and a third, dormant issue that may well re-appear after the national parliamentary election in 1991: whether to consolidate social insurance funds for health services into municipal revenues. All three issues have major implications for the type of planned market or markets which will eventually emerge, and we briefly discuss each in turn.

Hiltunen Plan

In November 1989, the Ministry of Finance released a one-man report calling for the replacement of the existing, national plan tied subsidy system for health and social services. Adopting a device which has been utilized by the Danish (subsequently phased out) and Norwegian (with an exception for child care services) governments, this Hiltunen Plan will create a system of block grants, in which national operating subsidies would be transferred to the municipalities with few if any stipulations about their use. Through a complicated set of funding formulas, the existing subsidy arrangement based on current operating costs for services will be transformed over a ten-year period into a considerably smaller subsidy system based only on the age-adjusted population structure within each municipality. This block grant system will include education as well as health and social service revenues, but in a change from the original plan, the municipality will not be able to transfer national funds between these two separate areas.

In the legislative proposals presently being drafted, it is not clear whether each municipality will be entitled to decide whether to produce a particular service itself or to contract out to a private provider – a freedom which would require the elimination of existing restrictions on the percentage of national funds which can be used to purchase private services. This aspect of the block grant scheme will be crucial in determining the future role of the private sector in Finland, and may reflect current levels of municipal dissatisfaction with publicly operated services. If publicly operated hospitals find themselves forced to compete for municipal contracts against private providers, a set of management incentives similar to those to be unleashed in Sweden in the Stockholm and Kopparberg experiments, as well as in the UK by the *Working for Patients* report, can be expected. Not surprisingly, some Finnish hospital administrators are already preparing their institutional informative systems in anticipation of what one termed 'the biggest change since the passage of the 1972 Primary Health Act'. However, there seems to be surprisingly little planning within the public primary health centres for the financial changes scheduled for January 1993.

One element of the current national planning process that probably will not change under the Hiltunen scheme concerns controls over capital expenditures. Much as in the prior national planning system, the national government will have to approve expenditures over 15 million Finnmarks (about US $4 million), while the provincial government will be expected to approve all expenditures under that limit down to 1 million Finnmarks ($250 000). National funding for capital expenditures will probably be controlled through a separate block grant arrangement. These continued governmental controls are intriguing given the degree to which the wealthier municipalities have already sidestepped the previous mechanism to ration capital construction.

Local planning officers

The practical ability of Finnish municipalities to exercise their formal responsibilities with regard to the planning and strategic management of health institutions has been heavily constrained. Faced with physician dominance over internal institutional information (to the extent it exists) as well as over decision-making agendas, the power of municipal health related boards, beyond rubber-stamping budgets, has been, in the words of one member, 'only the power to wonder' (Saltman, 1987). In this unsupervised environment, it is not surprising to find that some primary care physicians, citing the press of population-based responsibilities mandated by the National Board of Health, see few patients. In one health centre, perhaps as an extreme example, primary care physicians see patients for only 25 per cent of their working time.

In an effort to reverse this local decision-making imbalance, a Ministry of Social Affairs and Health working paper in summer 1990 discussed the creation of a planning officer for health services within each municipal administration. Moreover, to facilitate this new officer's activities, a nationally developed management information system is under study.

Initially, it is thought that this planning post could be a part-time position, perhaps filled by a health centre physician. Once the information system is in place, however, and it becomes possible for this officer to track not only planning information but also the pattern of current expenditures, the role of the officer may change. A key point reflects the fact that the Finnish municipalities must pay hospitals not only for patients sent by their own health centre physicians, but also for patients referred by private practitioners. Once the extent to which municipal expenditures are being driven by private as well as public referrals becomes apparent, so the logic goes, the planning officer will spearhead local initiatives to introduce effective management control systems for both private and public physicians. Whether this proposal is adopted in its present form, and whether or not this progression from municipal planning to management activities takes place as foreseen, the character of the proposal suggests that the issue of municipal management of health services will eventually emerge as a major health policy issue in the Finnish system.

Consolidating social insurance revenues

Despite the current climate of administrative consolidation at national, regional and local levels in Finland, there has as yet been little serious discussion about the advantages of consolidating the two separate public streams of health care revenue. Experience with a single financial source in Canada (Evans, 1986) and Great Britain (Ham *et al.*, 1990) has reinforced theoretical arguments about the efficiencies of creating one monopsonistic payer. Moreover, Sweden's 1985 fusion of a similar two-track revenue system has been deemed a successful cost containment tool by Conservative and Social Democratic politicians alike.

In the Finnish context a proposal to redirect social insurance revenues into municipal control will be particularly difficult to adopt. Its opponents are likely to include not only the Finnish Medical Association, which remains a powerful political force, but also the rurally based Centre Party, which set up and still controls the social insurance system. As a result, knowledgeable observers anticipate that this sensitive issue of financial consolidation will probably be taken up only after the 1991 national election.

It appears almost inevitable, however, that this issue will be pushed to the forefront of the national government's agenda by continued fiscal haemorrhaging of both state and local revenues under the present arrangement. As social insurance expenditures have increased in the last half of the 1980s, the national government, unwilling to raise already high labour costs by increasing the social insurance tax, has had to dip into general revenues. In 1988, the national government had to contribute 12 per cent of the national health insurance's operating costs (Kalimo, 1990). Moreover, the national government's concern about costs led it to ignore a 1987 commission report which proposed higher real subsidies for private sector medicine (Kalimo, 1990). At the municipal level, as already noted, the amount of public hospital expenditures generated by non-municipally controlled referrals from private physicians is likely to become apparent once a new health information system is developed. Much as in Sweden in the early 1980s, the pressure upon national and local politicians to streamline health care reimbursement in a single local authority may well become too great to resist.

In the present Finnish policy climate, it remains unclear whether the Swedish Dagmar Reform's additional role in extending the clinical purview of the publicly operated health system will become attractive. In the evolving Finnish context, it may be that the removal of existing restrictions on municipal contracting for private services, as envisioned by the Hiltunen Plan, could, if adopted, establish a policy environment in which private contracting could be expanded beyond Sweden's experiences to include not only current privately directed revenues flows but new public operating funds as well.

CONCLUSIONS

The present health policy process in Finland, viewed at its broadest, suggests that several different types of planned market models are vying for political support. Although future trends appear to reinforce the health care role of local government over the long run, how particular solutions will be designed – and by whom – remains to be determined.

Recent experiments and proposals could be interpreted as containing substantial elements of one of three planned market models. One, as represented by the original Personal Doctor Programme, involves the nationally designed and mandated implementation of a new planned structure for delivering services and compensating providers. In the first and second phases of the Personal Doctor Programme demonstration project, a measure of individual choice of physician and/or physician team (but not site of care) was combined with a modified 'market share' payment system constructed upon annually capitated and preventive outreach definitions of patient volume. In both phases, decisions on how to structure the market, which actors to incorporate within it and the design of specific financial and profession incentives were tightly controlled within the national planning process. Equally importantly, all revenue flows remained publicly generated and publicly managed within the delivery system

A second, quite different, planned market model is represented by recent decisions to 'melt' the national plan in favour of direct municipal control. The decentralization of public sector authority from national to local level, as envisioned by the combination of the new law on specialist hospital districts and the Hiltunen Plan, largely surrenders national planning control over the specific market-style incentives to be adopted. Two key issues will be whether the specialist districts or the municipalities themselves will be entitled to make contracts with out-of-district providers of secondary care services, and the amount of designated funds with which municipalities can purchase privately produced services. This second model may enable municipalities not only to shift clinical production priorities inside the public system but also to contract out specific clinical services to private sector providers.

Viewed analytically, the municipalities gain one type of market advantage through private contracts – flexibility in the hiring of additional personnel and in expanding expensive services – but at the potential loss of effective control over the incentives that structure staff working conditions and responsiveness to patients. In this second model, all financial streams continue to remain in public sector hands, although the locus of control has shifted from national planning to regional municipal federations or to local municipal authorities. In addition, clinical provision may well move from wholly public to a mixed public and private arrangement. Thus, the second planned market model involves a changed level of public sector authority and a different form of market-based incentives, relying predominantly upon empowered managers rather than patient choice, but it remains a wholly publicly financed delivery structure.

The third planned market model (although it was not perceived as such when it was introduced in 1964) involves the subsidized character of the private health care sector in Finland. In this approach, neither the national planning infrastructure nor the municipal officials play much of a role. Rather, the public or 'planned' element involves the combination of two national financial subsidies: from the social insurance system for privately delivered services, and from the Ministry of Finance in the form of tax deductibility for private insurance premiums (companies) and private sector fees (individuals). In this third model, direct public revenues comprise substantially less than the total funds involved, and public sector control over the market incentives incorporated into service production is indirect and limited.

This overview indicates a variety of unresolved issues which will affect the future of Finnish health policy. The ongoing development of various planned market models suggests that future policy options will increasingly reflect choices among three or perhaps more market-derived approaches, rather than a return to the prior centrally mandated national planning process. Similarly, the degree to which various planned market models may be complementary to each other, and suitable for simultaneous development within different sectors of the health system, has yet to be explored. Most importantly, the impact of these possible planned market models upon such crucial issues as continued equity in access to care, the quality of care and progress towards the stated policy objectives of the Health for All programme have not been fully assessed.

Despite its international image as a success story for centralized health planning – or perhaps as a result of it – the overall picture in Finland now reflects the same basic factors that are driving decision-making and policy within other publicly operated health systems in Northern Europe. Once again, there is a fundamental sense of openness about the proper direction of future long-term policy, and a growing experimentation with various forms of planned markets in an attempt to design workable new structures.

6

AN ANALYTIC OVERVIEW OF PLANNED MARKET INITIATIVES

The concept of a planned market covers a broad range of organizational territory. The specific health care objectives to be achieved, as well as the precise mix of mechanisms by which to reach them, can vary considerably, depending on political, cultural or normative preferences. Further, as in all policy questions, there remains the potential for unintended outcomes that typically accompanies implementation of a new initiative within the public sector (Pressman and Wildavsky, 1973).

The review of recent structural innovations presented in this book suggests both similarities and dissimilarities among the three Northern European health systems described. While each publicly operated system has its own internal organizational pattern, there are clear parallels among the types of pressures for change which each of them currently confronts. In response, each country has begun to develop one or more planned market models as a potential replacement for its previous command-and-control planning approach. Furthermore, despite the broad nature of the dilemma they confront, all three of these health systems have thus far opted for reforms that remain more 'reformist' than 'strategic' in overall orientation.

In this chapter, we pursue two different analytic perspectives on the policy issues presented in Chapters 3, 4 and 5. First, empirically, we briefly review the points at which the present health policy environment in the United Kingdom, Sweden and Finland appear to be similar. Second, adopting a comparative approach, we distil two basic or 'ideal-type' planned market models from current country experiences, which we then compare on a number of key organizational parameters.

AN EMPIRICAL ASSESSMENT

Present health policy pressures appear to be fairly consistent among these three publicly operated systems with regard to both intra and extra health sector issues. Among the most visible intra-sectorial pressures are those that concern organizational questions: the level at which to lodge administrative responsibility, the level for policy responsibility, and the balance between primary and acute services. Extra-sectoral pressures reflect the relationship between the health sector and developments in general society: the posture of the health sector within the national labour market, and the shift in patient expectations regarding public sector services. Each of these issues will be briefly explored in turn.

Assigning administrative responsibility

A predominant issue in all three countries has been the restructuring of the basic administrative arrangements through which health services are delivered. A key pressure, reflecting changes in clinical thinking, has been to integrate delivery of primary care and social services. In Finland and Sweden, recent initiatives have sought to combine organizational responsibility for primary and social care, and initiatives in both countries have sought to root this integrated framework at the local governmental level, in the municipality. In the United Kingdom, a roughly similar set of proposals were put forward in the 1988 Griffiths Report on community care (HMSO, 1988).

A second group of administrative issues concerns the fate of intermediate or regional level bodies within these three publicly operated health systems. Although there has been considerable discussion, the likely direction or outcome remains undecided. On the one hand, several recent initiatives and proposals appear to point towards a strengthened regional administration. In Britain, the 1989 white paper proposes to consolidate key remaining regional health authority functions (including supervision of specialist physician contracts and controls over capital expenditure) into the district health authority. In Finland, the national parliament has adopted legislation combining administration for more than 100 separate speciality care hospitals into 22 comprehensive specialist hospital districts. In Sweden, the 1983 Health Act gave the 26 county councils independent responsibility for the design and delivery of health services, and the 1985 Dagmar Reform consolidated the last separate health care revenue stream into the county treasury.

There are also many indications that suggest, more or less simultaneously, that regional administrative bodies may find their authority reduced or eliminated in the not too distant future. In the UK the 1989 working paper would not only transfer certain new responsibilities to the district health authority, it would also reduce district control over services through the creation of semi-autonomous self-governing hospital trusts as well as budget-holding general practitioners. In Sweden, where the county councils have provided acute services since 1864, there is continuing discussion about whether this regional form of health administration may have outlived its usefulness (Landstingsförbundet, 1986; *Dagens Nyheter*, 16 April 1989), particularly if the primary care sector were to be given over completely to the municipalities, to complete the integration of primary with social services (thereby adopting a Finnish model of administration). In Finland, the Conservative–Social Democratic coalition government proposed to reinforce its 'free municipality' experiment with a new block grant subsidy structure, in which national resources for municipally produced services will be given directly to municipal governments (the Hiltonen Plan), eliminating provincial (and National Board of Health) control over the allocation of health sector funds and personnel posts.

Assigning policy responsibility

Parallel to questions about the appropriate level of government to administer health services there have been debates about the appropriate level at which to formulate health policy. In the UK the ministry appears intent on gaining additional levers over national policy formation – beyond the existing centralized structure of the National Health Service. The 1989 white paper proposed that ministers retain discretionary 'reserve powers' to intervene at any level of the delivery system, including self-governing hospital trusts. Similarly, at least during the first year of implementation (April 1991 to March 1992), hospital trusts will be required to obtain Treasury Department approval for major capital expenditures.

Within the Swedish and Finnish systems, concern about the national policy role reflects reversal of a 20-year trend in which service delivery responsibility had been devolved to regional or municipal governments. Both national governments, reassessing their position on the trade-off between local synergies and loss-of-control in a decentralized system, have sought to consolidate existing national policy levers within their respective ministries of social affairs and health. In both countries, official consideration was given to restructuring their quasi-independent national boards of health (in Sweden, National Board of Health and Welfare) into 'planning departments' inside the ministry. These efforts were inspired in part by the perceived resistance of physician-dominated boards to the ministry's new politically generated policy imperatives. While restructuring was ultimately dropped in the Swedish case, in Finland a partial reconfiguration is underway.

The national ministries are also interested in retrieving certain policy-related levers from existing regional level administration. In the UK, where the Department of Health (formerly part of the Department of Health and Social Security) exerts central control over the NHS, the 1989 white paper proposed the elimination of local authority representation from district authority boards, further consolidating policy responsibility in national political hands. In the Swedish case, the national government has sought to compensate for a part of the policy authority which was given over to the 26 counties in the 1983 Health Act. Although the Swedish ministry's immediate concern has been to blunt popular dissatisfaction with high visibility issues like queues for elective surgical procedures, the creation of new nationally led policy institutions (particularly the Prime Minister's research committee and the appropriate technology office inside the ministry) suggests longer term policy objectives as well. The National Board of Health and Welfare, working along similar lines, has sought to carve out a new role for itself in evaluating the quality of county health care services. In Finland, official policy formulation thus far remains very much a national government function. Of course, while the regional (provincial or hospital federation) apparatus has no formal policy-making role, these bodies shared considerable informal policy-making authority within the structure of the national plan (Saltman, 1988a), authority which the new specialist hospital districts may well inherit. However, the ministry has reinforced its own authority at the central level by taking over direct supervision of the national planning process from the National Board of Health.

Balancing primary and acute services

An increasingly painful pressure upon all three publicly operated health systems has been the re-emergence of acute hospital services as a priority funding candidate. This is not surprising, since the rapid developments in intensive clinical care that lie behind this are international in character. The intensity of demand for new hospital resources may also reflect success, in Sweden and Finland, in directing funding towards primary care services earlier in the decade.

Increasingly important is the rise in popular resentment over inpatient hospital inadequacies and the resultant queues. Although queues for certain elective surgical procedures had averaged two years or longer in some districts within all three countries for some years, public outcry rose dramatically in 1987 and 1988. The combination of available new technology, public demand and previous resource rationing placed substantial pressures on British, Finnish and Swedish service providers to increase funding to their hospital sectors. As a consequence of this 'shift in the wind', funding for primary care services – despite protestations – may well be downgraded to co-equal status.

Recruiting sufficient personnel

Beyond intra-sectorally generated pressures for change, there are commonalities among these publicly operated health systems in terms of issues posed by the wider economic and social environment in which they function. While other economic questions may have received more international attention, one of the most aggravating external pressures upon all three health systems has been the shortage of trained nursing, social service and other middle and lower level professional personnel. In the UK the lack of sufficient nursing personnel has been an important factor in the inability of acute hospitals to reduce queues for elective surgery. In Sweden the labour shortage has forced some county councils to reduce services and close badly needed nursing home beds. Finland has begun to experience a nursing shortage in its larger acute institutions. In all three countries, the labour shortage is most acute within prosperous metropolitan areas, and in particular within the capital cities.

While nursing has faced the most difficult recruitment problems, similar personnel issues can be found elsewhere in the health and social service sectors in all three countries. In Finland health centres have faced increasing difficulty in recruiting and retaining general practitioners – a problem estimated as affecting nearly all of Finland's 200 health centres by summer 1990. In Sweden the counties have instituted a wide variety of initiatives seeking to make social service and home care work more attractive to new entrants to the workforce.

Viewed more broadly, current labour market difficulties in the health sector may well be the inevitable consequence of national macroeconomic policies in the early and mid-1980s. Confronted by a globalizing world economy, governments in all three countries (largely irrespective of party ideology) sought to shift resources from public sector consumption to private sector production (Bosworth and Rivlin, 1987). The 'success' of these macroeconomic policies – as defined by improved national economic growth – could be anticipated to affect the overall competitiveness of public sector human services in a tightening labour market. Indeed, the fact that all three health systems continued to experience nursing shortages despite the onset of the 1990–1 recession suggests the importance of long-term structural obstacles to a more effective labour market policy in the health sector.

Changing patient expectations

A growing external pressure is the demand by patients for more influence over the terms on which they receive care. Visible popular concern over issues like elective surgical queues has generated pressure to alter provider behaviour within all three publicly operated health systems. Beyond this prioritization issue, however, there is a growing consciousness among patients that they should participate more actively in decisions about the clinical treatment they receive and which particular site and medical professional delivers services to them. While these pressures are currently strongest in Sweden (Saltman and von Otter, 1987; Landstings-förbundet, 1991), the issue is gaining attention in the United Kingdom (Ham, 1988; Scrivens, 1988; Green *et al.*, 1990) and also in Finland.

This movement towards 'patient empowerment' suggests a considerable challenge to traditional planning rationalities within all three health care systems. In the past, health sector officials and professionals have sought to match service supply with a demo-graphically defined framework for demand. In the emerging environment, patients seek influence not only over when, where and by whom services are delivered, but also, in the desire for interactive participation in delivery decisions, over how services are organized. Moreover, in all three countries, the growth of private providers who can respond to these patient-generated signals provides an unmistakeable warning to public sector providers who are slow to alter their behaviour and internal organizational pattern.

A COMPARATIVE ASSESSMENT

The key patterns described so far focus upon questions of recon-figuration of administrative responsibilities, reorientation of service priorities, adjustments in recruitment policies and shifts in patient expectations. These organizational issues, combined with the broader economic, demographic and technological pressures ex-plored in Part I, define the overall context within which these three publicly operated health systems confront what is the common strategic dilemma. Despite the relative similarity of the funda-mental situation, however, these health systems are in the midst of adopting three rather different mixes of planned market mechan-isms in their search for a solution. Although the external stimuli have been roughly equivalent, the responses of the systems have been parallel primarily in that they are adopting the general outlines of a planned market approach, but not necessarily in the specific design of those planned markets.

One of the most essential distinctions between planned market models concerns questions of ownership and operation of provider institutions. Although the United Kingdom, Sweden and Finland all contain private health sectors in varying degree, they have had a tradition for at least a generation of public ownership of the vast majority of health care facilities. For these countries, consequently, one key planned market distinction has been between the broad concept of a 'public market' for health services, in which partici-pating providers are accountable to elected officials according to the usefulness of services to patients, and a 'private market' in which providers report to private share, bond or loan holders on a profit-making basis.

It should be noted that this ideal-type dichotomy does not include what some would call a third, intermediate category – namely not-for-profit organizations operated by religious or private community-based groups. This intentional absence reflects two judgements on our part. First, the major source of new health care organizations in Northern European countries continues to be for-profit in nature, perhaps reflecting the inability of not-for-profit organizations to generate the sizeable start-up capital necessary to open a modern health services facility. Second, experience in the United States (Gray, 1986), but also in the UK (Higgins, 1988), has suggested that once competitive markets for health services are introduced, the behaviour of the not-for-profit organizations soon strongly resembles that of their officially for-profit counterparts.

Recent debate over the advantages or disadvantages of a structural shift from publicly to privately capitalized providers has been wide-ranging (see, for example, MacLachlan and Maynard, 1982; Culyer and Jönsson, 1986; Jonsson and Skalin, 1986). In the following section, we contrast two ideal-type planned market models which fall on different sides of this public–private divide. The first model, which we term 'public competition', reflects the central conceptual premise that underlies a number of Swedish planned market experiments, most particularly those in Malmöhus County and in Stockholm County's primary care services. The second model, which we term a 'mixed market', is associated with the initial UK proposals for district authorities as set forth in the 1989 white paper (although not fully introduced in the first year of operation and not fully descriptive of the likely behaviour of fund-holding GP practices). This mixed market approach, however, also characterizes certain aspects of the Swedish Dalamodel in Kopparberg County, as well as one potential outcome of the Hiltunen block grants scheme in Finland.

Two ideal-type models

A 'public competition' model, as it has emerged first in the Stockholm experiments but now more fully in Malmöhus and Bohuslän, seeks to generate a public market restricted only to publicly capitalized, politically accountable provider units. The central agent of change is the patient, who, with his or her choice of physician and treatment site, brings along both institutional budgets and personnel bonuses. Providers who attract a larger number of patients earn a higher proportion of the pre-established public budget, while, as demonstrated by Södertälje hospital in the Stockholm maternity experiment, providers who experience falling patient volumes find themselves in financial and political trouble. Moreover, through bonuses to salary, public employees are directly rewarded for higher rates of productivity and efficiency.

A 'mixed market' model, as detailed in the *Working for Patients* white paper in the United Kingdom (HMSO, 1989) as well as – somewhat differently – in the Dalamodel adopted by Kopparberg County in Sweden (SIAR, 1990), creates a mixed public/private market in which existing and new privately capitalized providers can bid for contracts (in the Dalamodel for primary care patients as well) against present publicly capitalized facilities. The central agent of change is the manager (in the UK at the district authority; in Kopparberg at the local district board), who is responsible for overseeing the design, negotiation, award, monitoring and if necessary litigation of service contracts to various publicly or privately operated providers. Present publicly capitalized institutions are likely to find themselves engaged in head-to-head competition – what one of us has termed 'financial competition' (Saltman, 1990) – which, if lost, could in principle result in bankruptcy and closure. Patients find themselves dependent upon managers' good intentions and judgement to secure adequate and timely services. This mixed market model has proved both politically and technically difficult to implement in the UK – as evidenced by the outcome of the rubber windmill experiment as well as the British government's decision to postpone implementation of the model's more aggressive aspects. Implementation has been further complicated by the creation of fund-holding GP practices, which will themselves be in competition with district health authorities, and which may well adopt at least some of the contract-related behaviour of district managers. In Sweden, similarly, it remains to be seen whether the Dalamodel will in fact be introduced as designed.

An analytic comparison

Both public competition and mixed market models share central planned market objectives concerning the future of publicly operated health care systems. Each seeks to improve the internal efficiency with which necessary services are delivered and reflects a specific set of conscious choices about how to introduce market-style incentives into existing allocation-based management structures. Both models seek to utilize existing capital resources more productively, to make physician practice patterns more cost-effective, and to reduce the need to ration elective surgical (and other) procedures through unacceptably long queues. In the long term, both models supplement existing 'prestige-based' notions of competition among public providers with economically grounded incentives intended to transform the system's organizational culture and hence to generate 'strategic reform'.

The specific market-derived mechanisms utilized in each of these ideal types differ substantially. Public competition harnesses patient choice, on the demand side of the economic equation, while a mixed market relies predominantly upon competitive bidding by multiple (internal and external) suppliers on the supply side. The models utilize different actors as their major agents of change. Public competition empowers patients and, through them, concentrates incentives on physicians, staff and ultimately politicians to balance quality and price of care more effectively. A mixed market empowers district managers – acting as entrepreneural chief executive officers – to balance questions of quality and cost within their management teams in the search for less expensive forms of care. The two models also concentrate their efforts on different levels of the health care structure. Public competition focuses predominantly on changed incentives at the provider institution level – at the clinic – while a mixed market focuses predominantly on changed decision-making authority at the district level – in the administrative structure.

It is these three distinctions – the focus of economic change (demand versus supply oriented), the agent of change (patient versus manager) and the level of system change (clinic versus regional) – that define the essential boundaries between public competition as it has emerged in Stockholm, Malmöhus and other counties, and the mixed market approach developing in the UK and in Kopparberg County. Transformed into specific outcomes – internal economic efficiency, responsiveness to patients and political or normative accountability – these distinctions provide a useful framework upon which to structure the comparative discussion that follows.

Internal economic efficiency

In the mixed market ideal type, economic efficiency is linked first and foremost to managerial decision-making. The core assumption is that better performance can be achieved by granting managerial teams at the health authority (UK) or local district (Kopparberg) level stronger authority over both the supply (provider) and demand (patient) sides of health services provision. On the supply side, district managers are expected to stretch predetermined budgets through a combination of cost-focused contracting techniques and tighter managerial control over non-opted-out hospitals (UK) or local primary health centres (Kopparberg). Competition with private providers over district-level contracts will require major operating changes in district-managed institutions, including the introduction of various private sector mechanisms like case-based pricing and performance-related payment for personnel. In the formal proposals in both the UK and Kopparberg, district-level management is given substantial latitude over capital investments as well.

On the demand side, district managers will have enhanced authority to channel patients towards preferred providers. Beyond existing demand-side controls built into the traditional allocation-based delivery structure, district managers will have new authority to require patients to receive treatment from providers (whether public or private) who have successfully negotiated contracts with that district. Viewed overall, the mixed market approach thus emphasizes the role of broadly empowered managers to match supply and demand for clinical services, combining private sector style controls over health care providers with strengthened public sector style authority to channel and ration both the volume and the quality of available patient services.

The public competition model, by comparison, places only secondary emphasis on the capacity of managers to enhance organizational productivity. Instead, public competition as demonstrated in the Stockholm experiments concentrates on generating a demand-side or patient-led form of economic efficiency focused upon patient choice of service provider and site. Patient preference, based on logistical, quality and convenience criteria, whether at the primary care or the hospital level, triggers a coordinated pattern of budgetary and personnel-related incentives for improved clinic-level efficiency as well as effectiveness. This new structure of economic incentives is introduced within a defined framework of supply options, limited to publicly capitalized providers and by explicit political or normative commitments about the appropriate characteristics of service supply.

A major difference between the mixed market and public competition approaches concerns the potential impact of private capital on the operating behaviour of providers. The mixed market model, in its drive for supply-side cost reduction, creates direct competition between privately and publicly capitalized providers. To compete for contracts on a price-competition basis, publicly operated providers could find themselves forced to reconfigure both their organizational structure and their activities in the image of private sector facilities. Recent experience in the USA suggests that publicly operated institutions might well feel compelled to make substantial administrative investments to be able to cost out, price and market services. It is likely that public providers would also have to alter the mix of clinical services they offer. They could feel economic pressure to strip out the 'use value' (consumption value) aspects of their services, which in the past typically distinguished public from private for-profit providers; for example, preventive, educational, social counselling and referral functions. In developing new programmes, they could increasingly feel obligated to concentrate upon 'profitable' rather than 'needed' services. Viewed overall, the outcome could well be a 'levelling effect', in which public providers come to mirror their privately capitalized profit-oriented counterparts.

This levelling effect would have two major consequences for existing publicly operated systems. First, administrative as contrasted with clinical expenditures would rise dramatically. One often-cited review concluded that administrative expenditure in the pluralist USA health system, conservatively estimated, was nearly four times greater than that of the publicly operated systems in the United Kingdom and Sweden (Himmelstein and Woolhandler, 1986).

Second, in the long term this levelling of public and private sector differences could threaten the continued survival of the public sector as presently understood. Private for-profit providers have access to greater amounts of capital, in that they can merge or sell themselves to corporations with large capital reserves. As a result, they can more readily surmount expensive 'barriers to entry' in profitable lines of new medical activity. Private providers often have greater freedom of action to reduce short-term costs by lowering wages or laying off employees. Ultimately, if the private service sector becomes sufficiently well developed, it can turn the political tables and begin to question the non-tax-paying status of public and not-for-profit institutions – a debate that is well under way in the United States (Hertzlinger and Krasker, 1987). The final outcome from a mixed market could thus be that public sector entrepreneurial entities will not be capable of surviving in a competitive environment which is defined by and suited to the limited profit-oriented objectives of private capital.

In a public competition approach, the long-term outcome would probably be quite different. The absence of privately capitalized providers eliminates the potential for price-based competition to drive out quality-based forms of competitive behaviour. Public competition, as a result, is unlikely to experience a profit-driven levelling effect with its untoward implications for health system structure and behaviour. A variety of other, for-profit-driven difficulties related to efforts by lenders to dictate operating activities also disappear. But these mixed market problems might be replaced by the problems of insufficient or non-consequential competition. The combined interest of existing health providers, their unions and (in the Nordic context) publicly elected health officials, as well as the preference of some health care managers not to disrupt the existing organizational culture, may make it easier to establish the form rather than the substance of competition for public market share. It may remain politically difficult to introduce productivity-related salary arrangements for publicly employed medical providers or to link institutional budgets to public market share. It may also be difficult to persuade physicians to provide their patients with appropriate information and influence within the referral process. There is, finally, a danger that improperly designed incentive arrangements could convert public competition into little more than workforce speed-ups.

Responsiveness to patients

The distinctions between these two ideal types on the second major variable – responsiveness to patients – are complicated by differences in how the proposed planned markets would function with regard to primary care as against hospital level services. Although the UK and Kopparberg models both call for patient choice of general practitioner (in the UK) or primary health centre (in Kopparberg), they assign most (in the UK) or all (in Kopparberg) hospital-related treatment decisions to district management. The role of patients in these particular mixed market versions is considerably stronger than in a conceptually 'pure' approach, and thus the key differences from the public competition notions demonstrated in Stockholm County lie in their application at the specialist hospital level.

In the ideal-type notion of a mixed market, demand-related treatment issues remain under the close control of the district level manager. Patient concerns about the quality, location or convenience of provider services do not have independent organizational standing, but rather are to be incorporated into district management's overall effort to balance supply and demand for services at the lowest short-term cost. Although district managers are expected to weigh patient interests in this decision-making process, they will probably emphasize issues of cost since these are more readily understood by non-physicians. Moreover, managers' own performance-related pay is typically linked to expenditure-related definitions of productivity. In this distribution of authority, the patient has little or no countervailing power inside the service delivery structure through which to balance managerial decisions.

This minimalist role for the patient in a mixed market health system can be observed in the UK in the preliminary preparations for the introduction of the new system in April 1991. While district management has sought out general practitioners (often for the first time) and conducted patient satisfaction surveys in an effort to broaden service contract planning, patients will not have any effective means through which to modify or ratify a district decision about hospital services. Their only option, depending upon the procedure involved, may be to switch general practitioners from a district-linked to a budget-holding practice. Utilizing Hirschman's (1970) concepts of 'voice' (participation) and 'exit' (withdrawal), it would appear that patients in this new mixed market will, for hospital services at least, be required to rely mostly on 'exit' from the district-controlled system by transferring either to budget-holding GPs or to the private sector.

One potential consequence of the mixed market model's lack of emphasis upon patient interests (and formal empowerment) may be an increase in malpractice suits and recourse to other market-style forms of consumer protection. If economic pressures come to be viewed as altering clinical decision-making, a logical outcome could be that patients might begin to make stronger demands for formal rights within the legal system. With such a shift in perspective, patients might well be encouraged by the legal profession to file suit – an outcome which would be associated with considerable cost increases from liability insurance as well as, at a clinical level, for defensive diagnostic testing.

A public competition model, as demonstrated in the Stockholm experiments, takes a rather different approach to the question of patient influence. The central economic role of the patient ensures that the overall service configuration will be broadly responsive to patient-generated concerns about quality of care, logistical and convenience issues. This outcome reflects public competition's demand-led approach to the pursuit of economic efficiency. Moreover, the ability of the patient to influence where and from whom care is received, and the absence of profit-oriented providers, should minimize the impact of broader societal trends towards litigation.

The potential problems of a public competition model reflect quite different concerns. The degree to which a public competition approach empowers patient choice of providers and site suggests that certain barriers may be needed to restrict unnecessary utilization. Restricting patient choice of primary care provider to an annual selection period, like that used presently in conjunction with private practitioners' lists in Denmark, may reduce unnecessary costs. Such barriers, however, can exacerbate a second potential problem in a patient choice based delivery structure, namely the unequal ability of educated and better-off patients to 'work the system' more effectively. The ideal situation in a consumer-led market is one in which the more astute patients lead the way for improvements that benefit all patients.

Political and normative accountability

With regard to political and normative issues (equity, access and quality), a mixed market model presents certain unresolved questions. District management's central concern with economic efficiency in negotiating provider contracts implies several levels of potential normative risk, which in the UK may also affect budget-holding general practitioners.

Contracts granted to privately capitalized providers may, under cost pressure, generate below-average quality of care, particularly in service areas where professional medical interest is lower (Schlesinger *et al.*, 1987). To retain credibility in the supervisory process, a district or general practitioner may be forced to grant multiple overlapping contracts so as to have the perceived option of cancelling a contract for non-performance (McCombs and Christenson, 1987). Contingency plans should be developed to respond to unexpected provider bankruptcy or closure, such as the 1989 bankruptcy in USA of the largest for-profit health maintenance organization (*New York Times*, 17 March 1989).

Districts and GPs will also need to develop adequate (and expensive) mechanisms to protect patients from unscrupulous or exploitative private providers – problems experienced by private contracting programmes for Medicaid in the United States, in the early 1970s in California (D'Onofrio and Muller, 1977) and more recently in Arizona (Christianson and Hillman, 1986). Under even the best of circumstances, knowledgeable contracting for complex elective surgical procedures like coronary by-pass operations requires sophisticated analysis of hospital production information, often involving incompletely understood relationships between volume and quality of care (Freeland *et al.*, 1987).

There are, more broadly, potential problems inherent in district management's dual role as repository of both supply and demand within a mixed market structure. District managers supervise the publicly operated units that supply services as well as representing patient demand in the contracting process with privately capitalized providers. Given this dual role, it is unclear whether the district manager can be the disinterested 'sponsor' for patients that one theorist has proposed as essential to such a private contracting system (Enthoven, 1986).

Finally, a mixed market detracts from, if it does not directly impede, the ability of a publicly operated health system to pursue difficult long-term political objectives. By enhancing the role of privately capitalized providers, and by requiring publicly operated providers to emulate their private counterparts, a mixed market model serves to legitimate and institutionalize the existing process by which individual patients opt out of the publicly operated system. Rather than utilizing competitive mechanisms to improve the quality of essential public services so as to attract patients back, a mixed market introduces a version of competitive efficiency which further fragments the general population's relationship to the public system. Thus, one potential cost of a mixed market model could be the end of public consensus on the importance of universal publicly provided health services.

A linked normative consequence of a mixed market could be reduced emphasis upon the preventive, primary care based strategies for health system development promoted by the World Health Organization and accepted by its European member states in the 1984 target document (WHO, 1984). Experience in the United States has demonstrated that it can be difficult to retain health-related services once price-based competition for the delivery of curative medical services is allowed to predominate (Gray, 1986). Finally, it may be difficult and disruptive to coordinate the profit-oriented planning and delivery behaviour of medical providers with the client-oriented planning and delivery behaviour of social, educational and other publicly administered human services.

The political and normative ramifications of a public competition approach are more difficult to divine, partly because existing experience with it is partial and experimental. The normative characteristics of this model's decision-making process would, of course, reflect the central role of its participants. Planning activities for new services would, under public competition, remain a responsibility of public officials and thus continue as a publicly accountable rather than a corporate strategic endeavour. Service delivery would continue to be organized on a 'social contract' rather than a 'legal contract' basis, with all providers subject to public scrutiny and accountability. National model contracts for the purchase and sale of clinical services could be developed, with suitable quality safeguards, without risking contravention of European Community prohibitions against industrial monopolies. Operating and capital budgets would continue to be public information – available for academic inquiry and research – rather than proprietary information available only under stringent controls. Perhaps most importantly, patient access to care would continue to be based upon individual condition, rather than subject to restrictive budgetary devices such as vouchers.

The attainment of these normative outcomes remains politically contingent. Although patients would participate directly in the structuring of the care delivery process, decisions to prioritize specific clinical services would remain political decisions as they are now. While this outcome reflects the continuing role of publicly accountable authorities, it does not make selection among competing public needs less arduous.

Summarizing the differences

Although both ideal-type models would move publicly operated systems from their present command-and-control oriented administrative structure, they appear to do so in different directions and with a different mix of market and planning components. While public competition emphasizes the introduction of market-oriented incentives into the *demand* for health services, a mixed market approach concentrates upon generating market incentives in the *supply* of available services and service providers. While public competition foresees a future publicly operated health system in which relatively tight public responsibility will be maintained over the *production* of clinical services, a mixed market strengthens public sector control over the *consumption* of care. While public competition would encourage *existing* publicly operated providers to improve their overall performance, a mixed market approach would stimulate the entry of *new* privately financed providers into the health care marketplace. Related to this difference in economic methodology, each ideal type takes a rather different perspective on the other two differentiating variables – responsiveness to patients, and political and normative concerns – as well. While public competition seeks to empower *patients*, a mixed market would empower district *management*. While public competition would retain direct public political accountability for access and equity concerns, a mixed market seeks to insulate large segments of service delivery decision-making from direct political influence.

To return to the theme raised in Chapter 2, these two ideal-type models make different political choices about the type of planned market model they wish to create. They emphasize different market-based incentives, to different health system actors, and to a rather different objective purpose. The fact that both proposals call for the introduction of market-style behaviours in the provision of clinical services within publicly operated health systems may be considerably less important than the recognition that they harness economic forces to pursue differently configured political outcomes.

PLANNED MARKETS IN PERSPECTIVE

The current movement towards planned markets in Northern European health systems can be viewed as promising yet erratic. It is promising in that publicly operated health systems are no longer beholden to what has become an obsolescent command-and-control planning paradigm, and that the social accomplishments of these systems – such as establishing universal access to medical services – are more likely to be sustained in the future. It is also promising in that experiments and proposals for change are proliferating, and that the process of generating a new replacement paradigm is well underway. Yet the present process is erratic in that experiments have often been patched together quickly, without adequate consideration for potential perverse outcomes. It is also erratic in the sense that many programmes are clearly partial, aimed at resolving short-term dilemmas and thus unconnected one from another, and, as in the UK with the counterposition of budget-holding GPs to district authorities, occasionally creating new internal health sector contradictions and dilemmas.

While at the moment promise continues to override erraticism, the success of the overall enterprise will be increasingly tied to the design of more sophisticated and comprehensive planned market models, better capable of consolidating existing achievements in a stable and sustainable form. In particular, as demonstrated by the potential dichotomies that separate a mixed market from a public competition framework, it is essential that centre and left-of-centre political parties carefully assess the likely long-term social and normative consequences of various planned market models before adopting them for use.

The discussion of the Stockholm experiments suggests that the concept of public competition needs further development if it is to withstand critical scrutiny. How will the patient become an equal partner with the politicians in steering the structure and operation of public health services? How should individual provider institutions and clinics be organized to ensure that they respond to productivity as well as patient-generated concerns? What type of operating and capital budgets should be developed? How can the concerns of health sector employees, particularly lower echelon workers like those in home care and other social services, be addressed without inappropriately restricting the influence of patients and politicians? These and many other dilemmas remain to be resolved if the relatively new concept of public competition is to be able to compete in the long run with more traditional concepts like mixed markets or even fully privatized models. In Part II, we seek to provide both a theoretical and a practical framework upon which efforts to develop public competition can build.

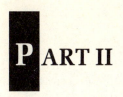

PART II

THE CASE FOR PUBLIC COMPETITION

INTRODUCTION TO PART II

Strategic reform in publicly operated health systems is a compli-cated and sensitive undertaking. As in other large but loosely integrated organizations, it is easier to identify problems than to achieve consensus about how to rectify them. Moreover, because publicly operated health systems are politically accountable agen-cies, the decisions they take carry implications for the future not only of health professionals, managers and patients but also of sitting politicians. To be viable, therefore, proposed solutions need to be not only clinically, structurally and managerially feasible but also politically palatable.

In this second part of the book, we develop a planned market model which we believe can address key normative and political as well as economic, demographic and technological challenges that confront publicly operated health systems. We begin by exploring two essential dimensions of strategic reform as it relates to the organization of health services. In Chapter 7 we argue that an overall objective should be to stimulate the development of 'civil democracy', so that citizens have greater opportunities to influence directly the conditions under which they receive health and medical care. We then examine in Chapter 8 the difficulties involved in delivering medical and social services at the local level, concluding that the existing administrative framework should be redesigned to incorporate an interactive relationship, within which patients and clients can directly participate in the design and delivery of the services they receive.

Following upon this conceptual approach to generating increased patient influence over the service delivery process, we develop in Chapter 9 a planned market model which can incorporate these broad principles into a practical and readily adoptable format. This model, which we term 'public competition', establishes a patient-driven form of market behaviour in which existing publicly capitalized providers are obligated by budgetary requirements to restructure themselves into 'public firms' capable of competing for 'public market share'. With this approach, we argue, publicly operated health systems in Northern Europe and elsewhere can achieve increased efficiency and productivity without surrendering their traditional normative principles based on universal access to appropriate care. In the concluding chapter, we summarize the arguments for the development of publicly capitalized rather than mixed public and private models of strategic health system reform, emphasizing the issues of responsibility and accountability within the dynamic process that will inevitably accompany the introduction of a planned market in health services.

7

CIVIL DEMOCRACY: A FOUNDATION FOR HUMAN SERVICE DELIVERY

In the modern welfare state, democratic theory has involved increasing opportunities for formalized participatory influence over three major aspects of modern institutional life: (1) over political institutions, via elections, party consultation with organized interest groups, etc.; (2) over social institutions, particularly pensions and social insurance against disability, unemployment, etc.; (3) over economic institutions, via industrial unions and forms of worker codetermination. What welfare state democracy as presently practiced typically does not include is formal participatory influence (4) over civil institutions, namely residence-related human services such as health care, education and child care. Although labour unions and left-of-centre political parties have placed major emphasis upon the transformation of political, social and economic life, they have traditionally viewed changes that increase the direct influence of the individual as a consumer of human services with trepidation (A. Martin, cited in de Faramond *et al.*, 1982). Reflecting this hesitation, the welfare state continues to allow individuals little formal authority over the residence-based institutions that in the twentieth century compose an increasingly important segment of what nineteenth-century idealist philosophers referred to as 'civil society'.

This notion can also be understood in pragmatic organizational terms. Within public-like private organizations, the importance placed upon attaining particular goals, and the interests served by the goals selected, reflect an intricate pattern of internal and external decision-making power (Crozier, 1964). Whether publicly accountable or market-driven, large organizations contain inherent pressures to pursue their own internal objectives and self-interest in lieu of meeting what are diverse and often diffuse consumer needs. Civil democracy, as we argue below, becomes a necessary corrective to empower individuals, enabling them to redress the decision-making balance within public human services.

In this chapter, we begin with a brief review of prior efforts to reorientate the administrative framework for public human services. Subsequently, we reconceptualize the core assumptions that underlie earlier reform attempts as a prelude to presenting an alternative theoretical analysis upon which to ground organizational change in public sector human services generally.

EFFORTS AT PARTICIPATORY REFORM

A variety of reform measures have been proposed or undertaken with the aim of reshaping public sector human service administration in Northern Europe. While these efforts reflect the differing concerns of their proponents, the intended objectives typically include at least formal interest in making the existing administrative apparatus more responsive to the public being served. In this section, we describe two different frameworks which suggest the conceptual dimensions of previous administrative approaches to enhancing popular participation.

One technique for restructuring public sector administration, discussed particularly within Nordic countries, has been to introduce cooperative self-managed forms of service provision. The intended purpose was to replace local level bureaucracies with self-governed organizations which could form a parallel power and delivery structure at the municipal and sub-municipal level. The preferred mechanism suggested to achieve this outcome has typically been to incorporate the general citizenry directly into the local decision-making process (Andersson *et al.*, 1976). This approach to system reform reflects earlier traditions of the social democratic movement based upon the concepts of guild socialism as developed during the early twentieth century by the Fabians in England (Cole, 1920).

A second approach to increasing citizen involvement in the design and delivery of community-based services has involved efforts directly to restructure local government and the lines of programme responsibility inside the existing administrative apparatus (Regeringens skrivelse 1984/5, p. 202). In this type of reform, local district boards are encouraged to integrate public sector services horizontally at the same level at which services are delivered, thus replacing what typically has been a functional organization on a separate programme basis (SOU, 1985, p. 28; Eklund and Kronvall, 1988).

The underlying objective in both types of reform has been to shift local decision-making responsibility within the existing administrative apparatus to a new participatory body, reflecting an explicit concern with reinvigorating public interest and participation in daily administrative life. The central objective is to invigorate local politics and the political party apparatus by empowering citizens as non-experts at the expense of appointed official and professional experts. At various stages within the different countries, reform has been championed by both conservative and social democratic parties alike. By reconstructing the existing political and administrative machinery, these efforts have sought to generate an intra-organizational counterbalance to what has been recognized as the overwhelmingly supply-side orientation of most public sector human services.

Viewed analytically, these and other recent proposals can be interpreted as efforts to supplement the representative democratic power of regular elections with the participatory democratic power of direct local activity inside the decision-making apparatus. This attempt to shift from the distributionist notion of substantive democracy to a more directly process-oriented participatory concept of democratic decision-making has important conceptual implications not only for residence-tied human services but for the objectives of the welfare state generally. Before we explore these implications, it may be useful first to consider the underlying theoretical premises upon which these and similar reform proposals are based.

ON THE LIMITATIONS OF VOICE

Using Hirschman's notions about exit, voice and loyalty (Hirschman, 1970), and above-described proposals for change rely in their essential components upon what Hirschman termed *voice* – raising disagreements with organizational policy as a member from inside the system. As a call for reform from within, voice has fundamentally different characteristics from the alternative active response which Hirschman posited – that of withdrawal from the organization or *exit*. Most importantly, voice involves a commitment to remain within the organization even if it ultimately does not change – hence Hirschman's notion of *loyalty*, which becomes an important threshold to the use of exit (Stryjan, 1989).

Evaluated as expressions of voice, the above-described reform mechanisms have strengths and weaknesses typical of this approach. On the positive side, voice-oriented reforms preserve organizational continuity and coherence, guaranteeing the continued importance of the existing decision-making apparatus in future allocations of authority and responsibility. Moreover, by retaining the existing organizational structure, voice can be seen to be consistent with the universality essential to the concept of equity within distributionist welfare state programmes. It encourages the individual to see his or her own needs and wants in a broader social perspective, and if dissatisfied to pursue not solely personal advantage but rather changes that would benefit all those similarly disadvantaged. These characteristics have often been viewed by labour and social democratic parties in Northern Europe as instrumental in creating social cohesion, a degree of classlessness and the attainment of certain collective goods.

On the negative side, one can point to a number of class-tied resources which are necessary for the successful exercising of voice. Those with better education, better self-presentation, and better rhetorical and organizational skills are more likely to find voice an effective option (Miller, 1988). Further, the individual requires unencumbered time to participate and thus, separate from issues of social class, the individual's ability to exercise voice properly is directly inverse to the number of arenas in which his or her voice is necessary. Perhaps most damagingly, voice alone can lead to passivity and to the fear of punishment if the effort at reform fails (Birch, 1975), a result which Barry (1974) terms 'silent non-exit'. This pattern of withdrawal from politics tends to be both cumulative and selective (Kavanagh, 1972).

The alternative which Hirschman posits – exit – has traditionally been rejected by welfare state proponents as being in fundamental conflict with the central public character of the modern welfare state. In the context of public sector human services, exit has been viewed as directly associated with expensive private-sector providers, thus placing the exit option beyond the reach of less well-off individuals. As the voice-oriented reform proposals imply, suitable models of change are typically seen as those that reinforce rather than dismantle the existing universal character of public human services.

Unintentionally, this exclusive emphasis by welfare state proponents upon voice has served to validate exit as the only effective alternative, and thus to legitimate Hirschman's conceptualization of organizational change. Recent proposals for change from left-of-centre parties do not consider the utility of what could be termed *lateral re-entry* – that is, the notion of partial withdrawal followed by re-entry elsewhere inside the boundaries of the public service sector. By presuming that an option to leave one's immediate service provider is tantamount to leaving the entire public system, existing reform proposals close off alternatives beyond voice that fall short of complete exit. In what is an ironically dialectical outcome, this insistence upon centripedal cohesion has introduced inexorable pressures for the centrifugal dissolution of the public sector human service sphere.

ON CHOICE AND CIVIL DEMOCRACY

The above analysis of voice-oriented reform proposals suggests that the present definition of welfare state democracy needs to be broadened. While past expansion from a predominantly political understanding of democracy has generated increased opportunity for formalized participatory influence over several major areas of modern post-industrial society, an important conceptual gap remains with regard to publicly provided human services.

First and foremost, democracy as formally defined involves direct public control over *political institutions*, via elections, party consultation with organized interest groups and the various official instruments of public policy formation (Lively, 1975). The social democratic vision of democracy, however, has traditionally extended beyond formal participation in political activities to providing guarantees that ensure equality of individuals in the control and distribution of key economic resources. Hence the practice of democracy has increasingly included direct public influence over

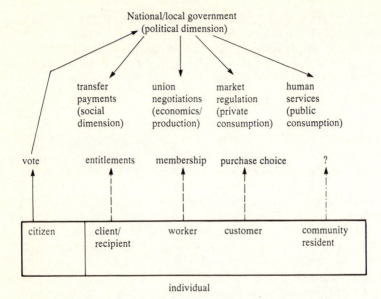

Figure 7.1   Constituent components of Swedish welfare democracy: a process model.

economic institutions – via industrial unions and worker codetermination; over *social institutions* – particularly pensions and social insurances against disability, unemployment etc.; and over *private commodities*.

With minimal exceptions, what welfare state democracy as presently practised does *not* include is the direct participatory influence of individuals over residence-related human services such as health care, education and child care. In the existing system, there is no equivalent act of individual validation for human services that parallels voting in elections, accepting entitlement dispersements, joining or participating actively in a union, or purchasing a consumer durable. The dilemma of civil democracy within the modern welfare state reflects the fact that one has been empowered as a citizen in political life, and as a recipient of entitlements in social life; one is at least struggling to be empowered as a worker in economic life and as a consumer of private sector commodities; yet one remains all but powerless as a community resident with regard to publicly provided human services (Ham, 1988; Petersson *et al.*, 1989).

Some proponents of the existing model of human services delivery defend this lack of direct individual influence on both theoretical and political grounds. Drawing upon a broad body of writings about substantive or content democracy and the importance of 'public good' and 'public commons' arguments, traditional social democratic theorists argue that only a mandated framework of equal conditions of human services like health and education can ensure proper development of a just society (Castles, 1978; Korpi, 1978). Criticism about the level of individual influence is deflected by pointing towards the multiple opportunities within the centrally administered structure to exercise voice from inside the system. On more practical grounds, proponents point to the obvious achievements of the existing system in raising overall living standards, particularly within the Nordic countries, and to the enormous difference between the situation of what can be termed the 'children of the welfare state' and that of those in the generations that preceded them (Erikson and Åberg, 1987).

The legitimacy of mandated equality of social conditions – of content forms of democracy – as against participatory influence in social decision-making – or process forms of democracy – has an extensive and often acrimonious history within Western political philosophy (Wolin, 1960). A well-known example is the long debate over Rousseau's *Social Contract* concerning the proper role of the 'legislator' with regard to the 'general will', and the degree to which it is justifiable to 'force people to be free' (Cassirer, 1954). These and similar questions remain at the heart of equivalent modern-day debates in Europe (Plant *et al.*, 1980; von Otter, 1991).

The distinction between content and process forms of democracy can be viewed as reflecting different concepts of freedom. Content democracy, from this perspective, can be logically associated with what could be termed 'freedom-through'; that is, the German idealist notion that the individual obtains the central elements of freedom in and through the social group – in and through society. Process democracy, on the other hand, can be taken as implying 'freedom-from'; that is, the Lockean notion that the individual gains freedom in separation from and often in opposition to the demands of other individuals. Pursuing a related analytic line, Berlin has suggested that there are both negative and positive components of freedom. One must have not only freedom from imposed restrictions, but also the resources necessary to choose and act (Berlin, 1969). Based on the assumption that a human is a social being, positive freedom can include many factors that influence his or her formation and can legitimate government activity to protect the individual from 'false conciousness', be it as member of the working class or as a consumer of public sector services.

In the present-day welfare state context, the appropriateness of continuing to maintain a predominantly content as against process model of decision-making for publicly provided human services can be questioned on pragmatic economic and political as well as theoretical and ideological grounds. A key economic argument is based on the contrast between the minimal nature of individual influence over publicly provided services and the mechanisms available on the private sector side of personal consumption. In most industrialized societies, private commodities are subject to indirect individual influence in the form of general governmental regulation concerning quality, labelling and safety. This type of influence is exercised through the electoral system. Yet in the case of private commodities, this highly indirect form of political influence is supplemented by a direct individually wielded instrument: the choice of the individual to buy a particular product from a particular manufacturer. As a consequence, the specific production decisions of the private sector, and the assumptions about individual needs and preferences that influenced those decisions, are subjected to an explicit process of individual validation, or, if one prefers a more cynical view of supplier-dominated market behaviour, at least of serial ratification.

Given the (occasionally incorrect) presumption of a real market with multiple independent suppliers of qualitatively different products, individual validation serves to ensure that there is an adequate fit between actual production and personal consumption decisions. It is not necessary to adopt the notions of radical-right economists (Friedman and Friedman, 1981), or to accept their trivialization of 'public needs' as only illegitimate forms of 'individual wants', to recognize the fundamentally different levels of individual impact on the internal behaviours of the private and public sectors.

A second economic criticism of the substantive as against the participatory view of the individual's relationship to publicly provided human services concerns the shift in the type of services – in the economic products – that the modern welfare state produces. Certain areas of state production continue to involve collective consumption in much the same way as they have since the 'nightwatchman state' of the eighteenth century, such as public safety and external defence, or, as in the early days of the emerging welfare state, services directly related to the bare necessities of life. Yet the human services provided by the modern welfare state involve the production of individually consumed services that cannot be as readily standardized (OECD, 1987). Public services now touch upon lifestyle-related values that are difficult to derive from democratic or general welfare-related social theories, but are founded in individual preferences, experiences and resources (von Otter, 1988). This major shift in the nature of public production reinforces the importance of reconsidering the mechanisms of individual influence upon service content and delivery. Increased citizen influence is particularly important in the health sector, where recent developments in medical technology pose numerous ethical challenges that can only be resolved on a case-by-case basis.

THE CASE FOR CHOICE

The political questions that can be raised concerning substantive democratic notions of human service provision revolve around the differences between choice or lateral re-entry on the one hand, and voice on the other. As noted above, choice among alternative public sector human services has previously been rejected as tantamount to exit and thus politically unacceptable. Yet in the present welfare state context, there is a strong argument that the most effective mechanism for enhancing individual influence over the array of residence-tied human services – for generating civil democracy – is that of lateral re-entry within the existing publicly operated service system.

Choice within the public – as opposed to the private – sector is only minimally dependent upon an individual's personal (class-tied) resources. One need not argue or organize others persuasively; find sufficient time or prioritize among competing participatory areas; or fear that sitting authorities will dismiss one's service preferences as secondary to other intra-organizational or political imperatives. Most importantly, one need not practice 'silent non-exit' out of concern for subsequent bureaucratic retribution. Instead, relying upon one's right of lateral re-entry, one can simply take one's custom elsewhere in the public sector.

Viewed from the present Northern European perspective, with

its existing highly articulated human services structure, publicly delimited choice would be a more egalitarian mechanism of individual influence than voice. Indeed, in seemingly logical contradiction, the realistic opportunity to exercise choice in the form of convenient lateral re-entry would serve to empower and democratize voice. Once individuals had the option to shift public providers – and particularly if public budgeting for service units reflected such shifts contemporaneously – human service organizations would undoubtedly become more responsive to the expressed concerns of their client population.

Similarly, resident and client associations concerned about quality of service questions would find themselves taken more seriously than they are at present in an exclusively voice-oriented environment. Indeed, adding choice to voice would create the structural pressure that is necessary to ensure responsiveness from the elected politicians and appointed officials who administer human services in Northern European welfare states.

The case for choice within the public sector can also be grounded in a philosophical argument about types of freedom. While exit can be legitimately cast as based upon 'freedom-from', the concept of lateral re-entry can be viewed as incorporating elements of 'freedom-from' within a broader framework of 'freedom-through'. In practical terms, lateral re-entry is unlikely to result in situations that pit the freedom of one against the freedom of others, or to damage the collective solidarity that has been the hallmark of content democracy.

There is, finally, a more general argument about the educational advantages of creating a learning environment that facilitates as much choice as possible within society. Numerous social commentators have observed that individual and associational decision-making increases the overall knowledge, confidence and ability of the citizenry. As Mill (1861) aptly summarized this notion, 'The most important point of excellence which any form of government can possess is, to promote the virtue and intelligence of the people themselves.'

CONCLUSIONS

Viewed conceptually, the exercise of public sector choice would add the validating aspects of process democracy to existing elements of content democracy. By combining a substantial measure of civil democracy with present opportunities to exercise political, social and economic democracy, the addition of public sector choice to community-tied human services would expand the existing framework of democratic life within the welfare state.

The public competition model that is presented in Chapter 9 was designed to facilitate the development of civil democracy within publicly operated health systems. Grounded upon the concept of public market share, this particular planned market model empowers the community resident by linking individual choice among (public) health providers directly to the short-term operating budget of service delivery units. Combined with salary-related and institutional incentives for internal efficiency, this confluence of patient choice and flexible budgeting would define a new administrative and managerial environment within what would remain a publicly operated health care system.

The adoption of a carefully restricted competition approach could provide a suitable means by which to pursue civil democracy within the context of the welfare state generally. Armed with the ability to exercise individual preferences reflecting service quality, convenience and effectiveness, and reinforced by budgetary consequences for service providers contingent upon the exercise of these individual preferences, the consumer would become empowered within the public sector delivery apparatus. Safe within a politically accountable public delivery system, individuals might well exercise considerably greater power in terms of achieving desired outcomes within this public market than they typically can exert within a traditional *caveat emptor* (buyer beware) private marketplace. Properly designed, competition can thus provide an appropriate vehicle through which to revitalize existing publicly operated health systems.

8

ADMINISTRATIVE RATIONALITY IN PUBLIC SECTOR HUMAN SERVICES

The dilemmas that confront publicly operated health systems reflect deeply rooted patterns of institutional authority and organizational behaviour within public human services generally (Weale, 1985). The preference for an allocative rather than an innovative planning methodology, the focus on input measures rather than output or outcomes measures, and the imperfect fit between services supplied by organizations and the services desired by individuals, can be found in varying degree not only in the health services but also in social service sectors as well. In important respects, the internal organizational difficulties currently experienced in health care mirror similar problems with the human service sector generally.

These dilemmas have become increasingly visible during the 1980s as a direct consequence of shifting macroeconomic policy within Northern European governments. Seeking to remain competitive in a changing global economy, ministries of finance have sought to restrict or stop the growth in national revenues consumed by public human services. For the first time since the Second World War, long-term trends indicate that expansion of the relative size and scope of public sector human services has stopped (Korpi, 1989). This shortage of new revenue has focused attention upon underlying structural issues, raising crucial questions about the future agenda of the public sector and the character of its internal organization and administration.

Most governments in Northern Europe have developed narrowly defined programmes to deal with various aspects of these public sector structural issues. While their proposals typically seek to achieve innovation, modernization and reorganization of service provision, different governments – headed by different parliamentary parties – have followed different paths to reach these objectives, with divergent roles for specific mechanisms like service privatization, service reductions and co-payment fees.

The re-emergence of structural issues in the welfare state debate was anticipated in various social science theories. Among the more prominent recently has been 'public choice' theory, a derivative of neo-classical economic thought that seeks to explain the behaviour of public officials and employees in the self-seeking framework of rational economic man (Downs, 1957; Buchanan and Tullock, 1962; Buchanan, 1969; Mueller, 1979). Organizational sociologists have also been critical of behaviour within public sector institutions. In a seminal critique, Crozier (1964) argued that large organizations suffered from a 'vicious bureaucratic circle' in which management parried each new attempt by employees to create discretionary work zones with correspondingly more narrow and counterproductive work rules. Perrow (1978) contended that sophisticated theory of any type – from human relations to the latest contingency models – has virtually no effect upon the inertial bureaucratic behaviour of public agencies.

From a managerial and administrative perspective, the most trenchent critique of public sector behaviour may well be Lipsky's (1980) argument that lower level public employees routinely break their own agencies' rules to accomplish official objectives regarding client service. 'Street-level bureaucrats' often spend their lives in a 'corrupted world of service'. From this bottom-up perspective, policy-makers can pursue two managerial strategies in response to perceived dysfunctional behaviour within public human service agencies:

1 Further automate, standardize and regulate the interpersonal interactions between human service workers and citizens seeking help.
2 Re-establish the importance of human interactions in the design and delivery of services requiring discretionary intervention or involvement.

THE LOGIC OF ADMINISTRATIVE RATIONALITY

Attempts to impose the first alternative – further to regiment human service provision – can only compound the organizational dilemma Lipsky described. Past patterns of human service development, particularly in the Nordic countries, have frequently been based upon 'rational' solutions imposed top-down using a social engineering model. This approach presumed that social needs were limited, universally applicable, detectable via available research methodologies and capable of being met by large uniform organizations (von Otter, 1983).

Three general strategies have dominated the process of rationalization in the public sector. They are:

● *Bureaucratic development.* Reflecting Max Weber's ideal-type model, emphasis is placed upon formal rules and hierarchical authority. Ineffectiveness is presumed to reflect employee discretion, thus requiring increasingly restrictive rules and tighter managerial controls.
● *Professionalization.* Proper training requires a theoretical understanding of the subject area. The formation of internalized ethical norms is an essential concomitant of training.
● *Technological rationalization.* Improved techniques of service management have influenced how certain public services are provided. Mechanisms include homogenizing clients, personnel and solutions to facilitate assembly-line production as well as an increasingly narrow division of work (surgery, catering, etc).

These three different strategies can be classified using two parameters, the level of organizational complexity and the degree of goal orientation. As indicated in Figure 8.1, bureaucracy implies a fair amount of organizational complexity (developed regulation) while professionalization tends to be more goal-oriented with (at least sometimes) less organizational complexity. Technological solutions often range rather high on both dimensions.

The extent to which a proposed solution is efficient depends on both the problem at hand and the implementation of the respective strategies. It is, however, a common fallacy to turn the relationship around and put the carriage before the horse: by implementing one of these strategies, politicians expect to reverse a vicious circle of ambiguity and managerial ineffectiveness. In reality, these strategies

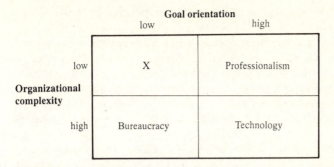

Figure 8.1 Strategies for rationalization in the public sector.

can work only when goals are sufficiently clear and effective remedies can be found.

Following this analysis, a core problem in human service provision is the balance between well-being as experienced by individual patients or clients on the one hand, and rationality as expressed by instrumental goal-oriented regulation on the other. Social programmes tend increasingly to disregard the former, viewing the client in 'machine-like fashion' (Habermas, 1981). This development is contrary to recent findings which indicate that human service organizations, to be instrumentally effective (to make people healthier, happier or cleverer), must give due respect to the well-being experienced by those they serve (Lynch, 1983; Waerness, 1984; Meldgaard and Andersen, 1985; Gough, 1987).

In Figure 8.1, a combination of a low level of organizational complexity and a low degree of instrumental goal-oriented behaviour is marked by an X. Organizational strategies based on this alternative can be labelled interactive, in that they seek to emphasize communication and contextual solutions in a type of 'ad hocracy' (von Otter, 1988). Conceptually, interactive organizations can range from informal close-unit family style relations to markets based on the supply–demand interchange.

PROBLEMS OF PUBLIC SECTOR ADMINISTRATION

Earlier studies (von Otter, 1986a) have demonstrated that administration of human services implies a permanent state of organizational ambiguity (March and Olsen, 1976). Similar structural problems do not appear in for-profit competitive systems, where individual or public needs are secondary to expressed demand, and where priorities over organizational direction are settled in terms of relative profitability. With a price attached to them, the values of service qualities like speed, convenience, choice and diligence become easier to distinguish. Moreover, prices provide a clear norm to compare apples and oranges, and thus dramatically reduce intra-organizational disagreement over goals, priorities and performance.

Welfare state politicians and public sector administrators are unable to use profit as an overall management technique in human services like health care and education. The determinative element in a public sector decision to produce a public human service is its consumption value to the citizen who receives it – its 'value-in-use' – whereas for a privately capitalized company it is the expectation of selling its production at a price which exceeds costs – its 'value-in-exchange' (Saltman and von Otter, 1987). As a consequence, the public sector requires a different, less explicit set of managerial models with which to evaluate organizational success.

This inherent assessment problem within public human services in turn generates a series of understandable but dysfunctional managerial dilemmas. The day-to-day operational consequences of unclear organizational objectives create what can be termed a 'vicious circle of ambiguity'. This self-reinforcing cycle contains two central components:

- *Ambiguous goals.* Reflecting the political logic that spawns them, public sector human service goals also tend to be amorphous and partly contradictory. Otherwise they might not attract a sufficiently broad political constituency to be adopted. Moreover, these goals tend to be derived from a general theory of needs – based on positivistic logic, rather than on individual wants. Yet real-world social remedies are difficult to establish and far less unambiguous than those derived from a technical context. Thus, human service goals naturally tend towards ambiguity from practical as well as political necessity.
- *Limited effectiveness.* Unlike technologically based activities, the organization of a public service can only rarely be constructed upon an effective methodology. The relationship within schools, social rehabilitation institutions, etc., between goals and likely outcomes, based upon the present level of knowledge and

techniques for education or social therapy, is only approximate and indirect.

Despite the ambiguous character of public sector goals, formal concepts of political democracy and public administration have traditionally required a sharp distinction between the political process of goal formation, on the one hand, and administrative implementation in the managerial and work process, on the other (Pressman and Wildavsky, 1973). As a result, a cyclical series of managerial problems tends to appear, constructed of the following elements:

- *Weak management.* Without an explicit hierarchy of goals and efficient means to achieve them, it becomes difficult to provide satisfactory leadership. As a consequence, most established management techniques for public human services fail. There is persistent unresolved conflict between limitless goals and limited resources.
- *Little positive feedback.* Public employees rarely receive an appropriate assessment of their personal performance. They seldom feel the satisfaction of knowing that they have achieved the organization's objective. On the contrary, tasks are often felt to be unreasonable and endless.
- *Irrelevant incentives.* Public employees tend not to be given meaningful and motivating incentives. The economic or social benefits they do receive are often not logically related to what is important in their jobs.
- *Ideological conflicts.* Management and field workers speak different languages. Unresolved problems related to the diffuse nature of tasks require impromptu solutions by employees' groups, without adequate managerial authorization or support.
- *Low work satisfaction.* Public employees tend to be less satisfied than other workers, and their work tends to become further routinized because of boredom. Work is not properly organized in order to maintain employee involvement.
- *Narrow divisions of labour.* Planning is separated from service delivery, and financial from operational management. Strong tensions between office administrators and field workers are built into the organization.

These problems reinforce each other in a cyclical fashion. Weak management leads to greater conflicts and fewer rewards, which makes management even less effective, leading it to increase controls and create a narrower division of work, which then increases problems of coordination and triggers off the next round of the cycle. In this difficult organizational environment, public sector managers neglect the special demands of organizations marked by ambiguity, with their special requirements for work roles, supervision, incentives, conflict resolution and patterns of interaction (March and Olsen, 1976). Employees, in turn, experience this organizational malaise at the individual level as feelings of burn-out and anomie, while on the collective level the result can be increased class-consciousness and union involvement.

In sum, the basic bureaucratic instinct to try to solve problems in public sector management through reliance upon power, control and more tightly defined work rules can only compound the public sector's organizational dilemma. In human services, moral ambiguity is inherent in the core characteristics of the job, and attempts to impose authoritarian solutions only exacerbate the central problem (Etzioni, 1988).

Solutions to this structural dilemma tend to emerge from the organization's informal authority system, often through collective action (Figure 8.2). Employees and clients (parents, patients, etc.) work out norms among themselves and resolve conflicts in a pragmatic interactive fashion. From the official perspective of top management, of course, this type of solution is unacceptable in that it violates the central distinction within public human services between politically determined objectives and their subsequent administrative implementation. Further, in some cases norms are established that are predominantly self-seeking, with little concern for the ultimate task of the group. Our conclusion, however, is that the public sector needs to learn precisely from this irregular 'bottom-up' management structure.

The organizational and managerial dilemmas described above can be illustrated by a practical example. Home care is a fairly new public responsibility in Sweden. It began in the 1960s as paid informal work for housewives willing to help an elderly or handicapped neighbour for a few hours per week. A cheaper alternative than nursing homes or hospitals, it soon expanded and the municipalities sought to organize the work more professionally. The introduction of professional groups was seen as making the job more attractive as well as increasing the competence of the organization.

Home care for the elderly started out low on both dimensions of

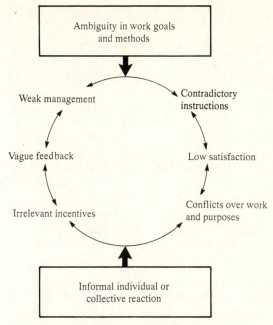

Figure 8.2   Public sector managerial cycle.

Figure 8.1. Initially, the work reflected typical characteristics of the informal sector within which it had begun. Employment relationships were informal and employees were paid by the hour without the support or benefits normally provided in more conventional jobs.

With increasing demand for this service – and fewer housewives around to do the job – institutionalization set in. Client well-being was operationalized into a number of separate functions. Rules and measuring techniques were developed, and standards for care, house maintenance and cleaning established. Specialized technologies were applied to provide efficient catering, bathing, foot-care and hair-dressing. Work therapy and paramedical assistance also became more professionalized. The results, however, were not what had been anticipated. Costs escalated and expected improvements in well-being failed to materialize. In their stead, feelings of estrangement and isolation were created (Gough, 1987). The home care worker now has less discretion over use of time, and the job is increasingly predetermined by structural boundaries generated by

'support' systems. Analytically, the following perverse consequences occurred:

● Multiple functions of various home care services have been
separated and assigned to different service categories of workers.
For example, preparing food can no longer be made into a social
activity between the home care worker and the elderly client
because no food is prepared in the home. Instead, an elderly
individual might be enrolled in a course in occupational therapy
where there will probably be instruction in 'therapeutic cooking'.
● Services are designed to meet a uniform need. These services are
unable to respond to individual preferences because of higher
levels of organizational complexity in the home care system.
● Specialized services are frequently provided in a collective setting. Those most in need of assistance, for example bed-bound
individuals, may receive less help, while the relatively active elderly are more likely to receive a full share of available services.

Overall, this dysfunctional outcome leads to growing frustration
with a frozen delivery system that meets official objectives but lacks
responsiveness, adaptability and coordination. At the bottom of the
emerging care hierarchy are still the home care workers, deprived
of their more rewarding and interesting duties, but confronted with
an uneasy client and unable properly to utilize their knowledge of
the client's wants and needs. One recent study concluded that participation in planning everyday chores is a 'social method in itself' in
relation to client well-being. It is not a precondition for therapy, it is
therapy (Gough, 1987). Other studies have demonstrated that
specialized division of work in health care tends to re-channel con-
tacts between the different professions or work roles through the
formal administrative hierarchy (Gardell and Gustafsson, 1979).
Contrary to bureaucratic, professional and technological notions of
rationality, therefore, a central element in improving home care –
like other human services – lies in creating new interactive forms of
public sector organization and management.

INTERACTIVE RATIONALITY IN HUMAN SERVICE PROVISION

The second policy response to the dilemma Lipsky portrays –
restoring the centrality of human interaction to public service

delivery – offers a more optimistic future to Northern European welfare states. An interactive approach to human service management would begin with both worker and client participation in service-related decisions. Their objective would be to define service priorities jointly, attempting to meet individual client preferences as well as the worker's professional objectives and responsibilities. Within the fiscal limits imposed by central administration, every client's care would be based upon his or her specific individual situation, reflecting his or her experiences, resources and preferences. General group characteristics – whether for patients, pupils or the elderly – would be recognized as insufficient measures of service needs. Consequently, each individual (or a family representative where appropriate) would be expected to participate in the formulation of problems as well as remedies. Most important of all, the design and delivery of human services would become an arena for recurring interaction between people, rather than a supply of fixed services. This is a critical change, in as much as well-being can only be created through social interaction.

Overall, the notion of interactive rationality connotes all factors relevant to individual needs that affect well-being. To implement this notion, an organization would have to deal with concepts quite unfamiliar to those versed in traditional organizational theory, including the rationality of caring, the importance of control over one's social environment and the experience of personal satisfaction (Waerness, 1984).

Reflecting this interactive imperative, human service agencies would have to recognize that organizational means and ends ought to reflect the context in which they are applied. The 'social competence' of the organization is decisive for its overall effectiveness and would be given a higher priority relative to 'technical competence'. The ability to improvise in search of creative solutions, reflecting 'local' resources, would acquire new importance, although professional knowledge based on generalized experience, as well as structured systems for employee monitoring and motivation, would remain part of the managerial picture. As a whole, an interactive, socially competent organization would incorporate the following three core characteristics.

1 *Democratic dialogue.* The quality of communication among managers, employees and clients is substantially improved, with particular encouragement given to the expression of qualitative or subjective views (Gustavsen, 1990). Management has frequent

interaction with the 'front', and seeks to facilitate horizontal communication among colleagues sharing similar experiences. Clients and workers are integrally involved in defining and interpreting key contextual factors that affect the quality of service delivered.

2 *Local definitions and decisions.* In contrast to traditional models of public administration, which postulate that politically determined goals can be implemented on an objective basis, an interactive model stresses the importance of subjective context in human service organization. Caring organizations require dynamic, contextual and complex patterns of reaction in which emphasis is placed upon teaching employees to generate solutions within specific client-related situations. In many cases, it is as important to know details of an individual's life history or immediate circumstances as to understand the biomedical causality of his or her condition.

3 *Individual and collective responsibility.* The need to integrate tasks and to pool resources implies that the employee should have considerable discretion in the work situation. But effective work also demands cooperation in groups, based on precisely the horizontal linkages that are difficult to create within a traditional bureaucracy (Tengvald, 1981; Svensson, 1986). To facilitate coordination in an interactive organization, all team members should be accountable for client-related decisions.

Constructed upon these three core characteristics – democratic dialogue, local definitions and decisions, individual and collective responsibility – an interactive organization would be better able to satisfy present day demands upon the public human services sector. Specifically, it could provide for increased organizational responsiveness to client needs; increase the quality of care through more adaptable routines; create better integrated professional roles; and build an organizational structure that contributes to the resource network around the client. Reconfigured in this manner, public human service agencies could adopt key elements of the self-managing team-based approach advocated for private sector industry by the human relations school of organizational theorists (MacGregor, 1960; von Otter, 1991). Returning to Figure 8.1, this new framework requires the reversal of developmental direction, away from increasingly hierarchical structures and back towards simple organizational models which can facilitate local and/or small groups control over client-related decision-making (von Otter,

1986b). It represents a 'controlled' breakaway from top-down bureaucratic accountability towards a more market-like relationship in which providers are directly responsible to the clients.

IMPLICATIONS FOR PUBLICLY OPERATED HEALTH SYSTEMS

As the Swedish case study illustrates, the generic problems involved in administering public human services can be clearly observed within publicly operated health systems. The inability of an organizational framework based upon classical Weberian rationality to resolve the need for moral as well as economic criteria in satisfying individuals' service requirements can be found at the more intensive, clinical, as well as the less intensive, social, end of the health sector spectrum. Moreover, the increasing importance of coordinating care across sectors (particularly from inpatient hospital to social service, and from primary care to home care) suggests that organizational arrangements that encourage direct horizontal communication between providers on an interactive basis will be essential to the attainment of normative, managerial and financial objectives throughout publicly operated health systems.

One major element of health sector reform emerges from the paradoxical outcomes generated by reliance upon a strictly technical form of administrative rationality. In the very process of achieving short-term managerial objectives, the health services undercut their larger purpose, which was to contribute towards the overall well-being of the individual who required care. In this respect, the perverse consequences of a programme's dependence upon a technical or rational approach bear a strong resemblance to the recent observation in welfare state theory generally that the perceived 'failure' of the welfare state in the 1980s reflects only the failure of 'technicist' methods and mechanisms of human service delivery (Mishra, 1984). This diagnosis, in turn, leads back to the solution indicated in the home care case: the need for a flexible interactive administration which can incorporate the individual citizen not as an 'object' but rather as the 'subject' of the services to be delivered.

The organizational issues surrounding the development of interactive rationality within human services organizations have important implications for the development of a new health policy paradigm in the 1990s. Just as a new paradigm should supersede the limitations of 1970s planning and 1980s neo-classical economics approaches, so too should it move beyond the managerial strictures of traditional public administration. If health service providers are to become more efficient, more effective and more responsive to patients, then previous managerial as well as policy imperatives will need to change substantially. In Chapter 9 we set out a planned market model which is designed to incorporate both types of institutional change.

9

A THEORY OF PUBLIC COMPETITION

Public competition involves the conscious introduction of a planned market for medical services inside a publicly operated health system. This planned market is similar to its private sector counterparts in that it is a dynamic process, in which specific organizational forms continuously evolve in response to changing conditions both inside and outside the health sector. Public competition is distinguished from a private market by the degree to which it can be held publicly accountable: under conditions of public competition, health sector officials retain the explicit responsibility to separate market signals from their usual consequences as and when necessary. The specific characteristics of this public market – the actors involved, the type of behavioural incentives, the linkage between operating and capital budgets – can be consciously configured by elected politicians to ensure that market allocation of health care resources reinforces rather than undermines the broader social objectives which form the conceptual core of publicly operated health systems.

While maintaining an overall commitment to social equity, a public competition based delivery system can help to accomplish three related public sector objectives. First, through its reliance upon patient choice as the mechanism of resource allocation, public competition stimulates a better fit between available health services and the particular needs of individual patients. Second, in its introduction of market-style signals about efficiency and effectiveness, public competition encourages existing publicly operated provider institutions to transform themselves into interactive organizations that can better respond to the requirements of their patient clients. Third, through its creation of clear incentives for health professionals and clear alternatives for patients, public competition motivates both the providers and the recipients of services to take more responsibility for the outcome of the care process. These three additional objectives suggest that a public competition based structure can produce improved provider and patient satisfaction while continuing to satisfy broader political objectives concerning equity and access to care.

This chapter draws upon theoretical aspects of public competition presented in earlier work (Saltman and von Otter, 1987, 1989a,b, 1990; von Otter and Saltman, 1988, 1991), as well as recent experiments in Sweden and Finland, to explore the administrative framework required to introduce full public competition at the operating level. Adopting an empirical methodology, we consider the appropriate design of a planned market which can implement public competition within existing publicly operated health care systems in Northern Europe.

AN OVERVIEW OF PUBLIC COMPETITION

We have described public competition as based upon three central tenets: (1) public ownership and operation of provider institutions; (2) patient choice of site and physician; and (3) flexible budgeting tied to public market share. We have also contended that the driving force of a public competition approach would be patient choice among public delivery sites and physicians for both primary and hospital care. Health providers, faced with individual choice, would be obliged to compete for patients – for public market share – in order to sustain income and staffing levels. While health delivery sites that attract a high volume of patients would be rewarded both institutionally (with more personnel when requested) and economically, delivery sites with shrinking shares of the public market would face contraction and, ultimately, closure. Finally, to improve the efficiency of provider performance, economic compensation and other provider incentives could be tied to delivery site efficiency, defined by compliance with some form of standardized physician practice protocols for common diagnoses in both primary care and hospital settings (Saltman, 1986).

The notion of patient choice that underlies this public competition model is rather different from that usually associated with the concept of 'free choice' in the private sector. Patients would choose among existing geographically dispersed facilities and providers, rather than between a number of competing facilities built close by each other in the same location. Although alternative choices would be easier to reach for residents of some areas of the country (in major metropolitan areas, or in towns located midway between equivalent facilities) than for those in more rural areas, the principle of patient choice would enable all individuals to pursue alternative treatment sites if desired. Given that the concept of choice reflects its own law of diminishing returns, in that having two choices is far more important (and more manageable) than having ten, the reduced number of service options in rural areas does not affect the usefulness of the central principle itself. In essence, public competition involves the availability of more than one option rather than an obligation to create a large number of entirely equal selections.

The planned market character of a public competition approach, particularly in comparison with the prior command-and-control planning paradigm, becomes apparent once we reconfigure the above description into the necessary practical operating components: (1) the centrality of patient choice in a new role as 'steering mechanism'; (2) the transformation of service delivery agencies into public firms; and (3) the design of a contemporaneous 'flexible budgeting' system based on 'public market share'. Each of these three conceptual components is developed in turn below.

Patient choice as steering mechanism

While patient choice would have a dramatically increased impact in a public competition based delivery system over its current role within publicly operated health systems, that impact would differ considerably from currently extant notions of 'free choice' as construed within pluralist insurance-based delivery systems. Beyond the important question of civil democracy raised in Chapter 7, this refocused role for patient choice would stimulate at least four separate, although linked, types of practical change at the provider level: improved provider responsiveness to patient convenience and service concerns; renewed health professional interest in structural aspects of institutional scheduling and waiting time issues; enhanced emphasis upon at least certain types of clinical quality; and – last but far from least – increased productivity inside provider institutions.

Turning first to the effects of fully enfranchised patient choice upon provider responsiveness to patients, health professionals would undoubtedly pay increased attention to such convenience and logistical matters as making and keeping firm appointment times, maintaining more flexible telephone call-in and appointment periods, and clearly explaining medical terms and alternative treatments to patients or family members. While these changes might appear to be minor in the overall service delivery scheme – indeed some planners and providers have been known to complain about the need to introduce 'charm school courses' – they represent the surface manifestation of a deeper shift in the process of treatment-related decision-making.

The second likely type of change, increased provider interest in the structural determinants of scheduling and waiting times issues, moves beyond convenience to more central questions of institutional priorities and objectives. Physicians whose earnings are dependent upon a stable patient stream – whether of new or repeat cases – are likely to express interest in inpatient or polyclinic procedures that affect patient scheduling. Matters from the relatively small (procuring computer software that will schedule fixed appointment times with specific physicians for a varying length of time) to more major institutional operating questions (longer hours and simplified booking procedures for operating rooms, greater availability of anaesthesiologists) will become important areas for physician input into hitherto essentially administrative or budgetary decisions. In effect, once health professionals' earnings become contingent upon their efficiency and performance, they will push their organization to expand its utilization of available resources.

The impact of patient choice on the third issue, quality of care, is likely to be equally valuable. In a public competition approach, patient (or family member) choice of physician and provider institution transforms the patient into an agent of quality control at the very heart of the resource allocation process. Patients or their families are likely to seek care from providers with the best balance of successful outcomes and acceptable waiting time, to the extent that this is discernable to non-medical professionals, utilizing available nationally generated information. While these decisions will be contingent upon a variety of factors, including the acuity of the condition, the availability of alternative sites or forms of care and the particular concerns of individual patients, these patient decisions will favour the highest feasible level of clinical quality.

Cynical comments by health system planners that patients will be seduced by physicians with the nicest smiles are contradicted by the same planners' fears that patients will overwhelm facilities that provide the highest quality of services. It should be noted that the exercise of patient choice, under conditions of public competition, involves patient selection among publicly accountable and publicly evaluated institutions, which would be required to maintain a high national standard of care in any case. In this context, patient choice has few of the dangerous 'buyer beware' elements sometimes found in pluralist insurance-based systems: in a public competition model, patients choose from among providers who satisfy prior clinical safety and appropriateness requirements.

The changed impact of patient choice upon quality issues can best be grasped by contrasting its likely outcome with those obtainable through currently utilized patient inputs such as patient satisfaction questionnaires. Unlike choice-generated preferences, which transform the patient into a central actor *before* the receipt of services, survey research data is typically obtained *after* treatment. Unlike choice-related decisions, which under conditions of public competition need not be defended through voice-based mechanisms, survey research results are 'evaluated' by professional providers who subsequently determine their relevance and usefulness for service provision. Ultimately, unlike choice-related decisions, which involve a form of participation in managerial decision-making and thus power sharing, patient satisfaction questionnaires are only 'opinions' which can be disregarded when they contravene existing producer-generated advantages or preferences. To be sure, quality-related improvements associated with patient choice inevitably and appropriately will be limited by many patients' dependence upon clinicians for advice, as well as by incomplete and occasionally insufficient information. Conversely, patient satisfaction questionnaires clearly have a valuable role to play in monitoring the attitude and performance of provider personnel. However, a public market based upon patient choice forces change directly at the core economic base of the delivery system, and is thus fundamentally different from a patient questionnaire approach that only addresses personnel attitudes at the periphery of the health care decision-making structure.

Fourth and finally, full implementation of patient choice would have a substantial impact upon existing provider levels of efficiency and productivity. Several of these outcomes are implicit within the changes detailed above: more responsiveness to patients, changed institutional operating procedures and improved quality of care (a crucial element in reducing expensive errors, the rate of inpatient re-admissions, etc.). However, the central productivity enhancement associated with patient choice reflects the consequences of clear professional and financial incentives for physicians and other health professionals as well as for provider institutions to increase their public market share.

Overall, the greatest stimulant to changed provider behaviour may be not the reality but the *possibility* of patient change, and the consequent *anticipatory behaviour* by provider institutions to alter their own practice profile so as to limit future vulnerability. As confirmed by recent behaviour among hospitals in the United Kingdom in reaction to the 1989 white paper, managerial changes in anticipation of projected structural system modifications may well be more substantial than changes observed after the formal change itself. Moreover, private sector experience in other industries has demonstrated that a small change in market composition – 5 to 10 per cent of the total – is sufficient to introduce major changes in the behaviour of both service suppliers and demanders (Porter, 1980). This level of patient change, one might note, indicates that only a relatively small proportion of patients need to switch for all patients to benefit. Thus, the introduction of patient choice within publicly operated health systems, even if it only generates a low actual change rate, can be expected to generate fundamental changes in the behaviour of health professionals and provider institutions.

As the Stockholm maternity experiment suggests, patients not only can have a substantial impact on the type and site of treatment, they can also generate pressures to produce organizational restructuring (the shared diagnostic services and closed ward at Södertälje Hospital) and, occasionally, changes in physician practice patterns (encouraging obstetricians to offer increased natural birthing options). One important aspect of the Stockholm maternity experiment which should be underscored concerns the key role played by patient information. The particular nature of the condition and patient involved created a well-informed consumer, with a variety of alternative sources of information (books on motherhood, peer group experiences, health centre midwives, etc.). Moreover, as is typically the case with elective but not acute conditions, there was adequate time to pursue and digest sufficient information to make an informed decision. Finally, perhaps as a result of the commonness of this condition among a certain age cohort, there were no apparent differentials in the utilization of patient choice associated with different social class membership or area of residence.

These characteristics of the public competition experiment in maternity care can be replicated in other sectors of the health, social and educational services to make the reality of client empowerment – i.e. the exercise of true civil democracy – meaningful. For example, in situations where fragile or vulnerable patients cannot make decisions for themselves, they could have a relative or friend serve as their advocate in choice-related decisions about health care – much as a parent already serves that function for a child. It also suggests that information clearing houses should be established in each service district to provide the knowledge necessary to make certain types of provider decisions. The clearing house concept has been utilized with considerable success for parent selection of public school in one Massachusetts city (Chubb and Moe, 1990).

A second point about the Stockholm experiment worth noting is that patient choice worked well without the need to establish either a system of vouchers or a network of negotiated buy–sell contracts for service provision. Rather, in the maternity experiment, the central county administrator designed a public market based on a fixed price for service (an annual capitated fee was utilized in a similar primary care experiment, increased to twice the standard amount for patients over 65). Thus, the new market was inexpensive to administer – it had low transaction costs. Further, individual citizens did not face denial of care due to voucher limitation or contract restrictions. A related example in support of a patient choice based market can be cited from Malmöhus County, where one hospital successfully utilized its ability to attract new patients from surrounding districts to preserve its status as a speciality institution.

The role of the public firm

A public competition model requires that important changes be made in the behaviour and incentives within provider organizations. Effectiveness in production obviously reflects more than the motivation and energy that employees mobilize at work. The structural character of the production process, the degree of vertical and horizontal integration within that process, the extent to which the organization can take advantage of large and small scale efficiencies, all affect internal operating efficiency as well. In traditional economics, this set of questions is usually discussed under the heading of the theory of the firm. To pursue the construction of a planned market, it thus becomes essential to develop an appropriate theory of the public firm for use within a health sector context (von Otter and Saltman, 1991).

In a public competition model, a provider organization ideally ought to have the basic properties of a firm rather than a bureau. It would be relatively free to design its own structure and make its own judgements concerning scale advantages, forward integration of production or market links with other stages in the health care production chain. A deeper understanding of the public firm and the trade-off between different levels and structures of integration could benefit from the organizational framework developed for transaction cost analysis (Williamson, 1975, 1985, 1986).

The effectiveness of an organizational structure in this analysis depends on two types of costs: production costs, related to the use of technology; and transaction costs, related to how relationships with suppliers, contractors, clients, financiers and workers are organized. These two basic approaches have been labelled markets and hierarchies: the former being based on contracts, the latter on vertical linkages. Firms traditionally try to capitalize on production costs by gaining scale advantages. More recently, they have also systematically pursued low transaction costs through negotiations and the conclusion of separate market contracts for intermediate products. There are both advantages and disadvantages related to vertical integration in a firm. Information overload, costs of control and difficulties in realizing synergies can cause high transaction costs. The large firm normally has advantages in technical, scale economies and transaction unit costs, but might have higher costs related to lack of flexibility and loss of control over labour. The trade-offs between production costs and transaction costs are often difficult to predict.

Coordination of production by means of the market – buying and selling – is an alternative means of management which is advantageous when information costs, capital assets and the risk of opportunistic behaviour are all low. One technique for avoiding certain risks but still enjoying the advantages of market flexibility is to adopt various forms of decentralized organizations. The multi-unit

(M-form) organization is seen as a transaction cost hybrid that takes advantage of both hierarchical and market characteristics (Williamson and Ouchi, 1981). Another intermediate form of organization is based on the distinction between hard and soft contracting. Under hard contracting each party is expected to remain relatively autonomous and to press its interest vigorously, while soft contracting would imply a closer identity of interests between the parties in which the formal contracts need not be as complete (Williamson and Ouchi, 1981).

In public services, planning has traditionally been based on the calculation of predictable costs, mainly related to production and capital investments. The more uncertain costs of internal and external transactions have largely been disregarded. The consequences are clearly seen in information overload, costly and inefficient command-and-control processes, inefficient contracting and exaggerated levels of formal integration. There is frequently a tendency to presuppose the existence of what actually has to be constructed, namely collective action. Yet the degree of cooperation needed for adequate levels of efficiency is reached not by presupposed harmony of interests but by the invention of institutions that produce order out of conflict (Williamson, 1975). The internalization of this presumption into microeconomic theory is highlighted by current arguments which move beyond the perception of the firm as a 'nexus of contracts' to an understanding of the firm in overtly political terms, as a 'nexus of treaties' (Aoki *et al.*, 1989).

Recent developments in the service industry have emphasized new modes of horizontal and vertical integration (Normann, 1986). Many corporations now choose to see themselves as delivery systems rather than production systems. A new institutional logic has developed in order to address the pre-eminent problem of complex services, which is informational overload of the organizational system. According to this analytic framework, functions are separated or tied together following social rather than technological functions. Similarly, firms try to become more efficient by decreasing complexity, by breaking off from the hierarchical order those functions that can work independently.

In the public sector, managerial prerogatives inside each new public firm regarding operating and production strategies could similarly span a wide variety of different managerial options. If, for example, an existing hospital or primary health clinic were reconceptualized as a public firm, it might decide to reduce complexity and overload by concentrating upon clinical services and purchasing ancillary and support services from other hospitals or outside vendors. Depending on the character of a particular service or product, a hospital might consider hard or soft contracting, or cooperation with other hospitals as an alternative to forward integration. Segmentation might also be adopted as a strategy to decrease complexity. An individual hospital might decide to address itself to a clientele with specialized needs in order to reduce complexity while at the same time extending new services to that group. Bundling, unbundling and rebundling are strategies that have proved useful in the service industry and that might be relevant for public sector health care organizations. Capital allocations could be split into two segments – those which demonstrably improve the operating efficiency of existing services and those which expand services or facilities. Allocations for the first could be handled by a public sector 'bank', leaving only proposals concerned with expansion for political determination. In short, once a process of creative restructuring has been initiated, public firms can respond with a range of strategic options to accommodate the continually changing environment they confront.

This notion of reconfiguring publicly operated institutions into public firms parallels two ideas that are receiving increasing attention in public policy debates in the United States. One is the concept of creating 'entrepreneurial government' by introducing a set of management-by-objective principles into the administration of public sector agencies (Osborne and Gaebler, 1991). The second is the possibility of applying the industrial sector theory of total quality management (TQM) to health care (Berwick *et al.*, 1990; Raimondo, 1991). Originally developed by Deming as a system of statistical process control for Japanese manufacturers, it approaches management as a customer-driven process focused on continuous quality improvement. Moreover, all members of the organization need to be involved, and there can be customers inside as well as outside the producing organization. This theory is constructed upon a number of the same core criteria as public competition: it is customer-driven and process-oriented. Public competition's central public firm framework could well benefit from similar techniques that generate continuous quality improvement.

Implementing flexible budgeting for public market share

Of the three core elements of public competition, the most difficult to translate into practice is flexible budgeting. With the exception of certain planned market experiments, public sector budgeting in most publicly operated health systems in Northern Europe still follows a fixed allocation approach on an annual planning cycle. Operating budgets for provider institutions are based on prior year allocations adjusted by estimates for inflation, utilization and new services (if any) in the forthcoming year. Institutional budgets, staffing ratios, capital budgets and personnel salaries are rarely contingent upon or contemporaneously related to performance indices such as patient workload, referral rates, operating efficiency or health-related effectiveness.

If patient choice of provider site and professional are to drive resource allocation, if patient decisions are to become a key 'steering mechanism' within public competition, public sector operating agencies require a rather different set of budgeting mechanisms. A new structure of personnel and institutional reimbursement is essential, in which the predominant component is each unit's ability to (a) attract and satisfy patients and (b) operate efficiently and effectively.

There is no obvious or intuitive basis upon which to transform the general concept of 'public market share' into a measurable and – for decision-making purposes, defensible – parameter of health system performance. What is required is a reconceptualized market structure that reflects patient demand but is not tied to a pure economically determined price mechanism. The objective is to establish a planned market that reflects the particular political and organizational patterns already in place within the host health care system.

Ideally, flexible budgeting for public competition should involve all three service delivery sectors within a health system – i.e. hospital, primary care and social services. However, designing flexible systems that can forge fiscal linkages across sectors so as to encourage treatment at the least intensive, but still appropriate, level of care is a particularly complicated process. Different sectors of the delivery system report to different municipal, district, county or regional governmental bodies, each of which jealously guards its fiscal and policy prerogatives. As a result, the introduction of effective flexible budgeting may well necessitate a system-wide strategic reform.

Public competition is designed to take place inside not only the *political* boundaries of a publicly operated health system, but also the *financial* limits of existing publicly planned budgets for health care expenditures. As such, public competition translates into a zero-sum competition among existing provider units for fixed, politically determined pools of aggregate capital and operating resources. Viewed in economic terms, public competition involves flexible budgeting for what remains a prospectively defined resource pool. It is *not* a system of open-ended retrospective reimbursement as in pluralist health care systems like that found in the USA. Equally important, as in all planned markets, the key precondition for well-functioning competition will be the clarity and appropriateness with which each existing health sector is divided up into specific zero-sum markets.

The size of a properly competitive market within each service sub-sector should reflect demographic as well as geographic characteristics. The goal should be to create administrative limits which accommodate 'natural markets' in terms of individual patients' preferences for care. Much as in the case of 'natural markets' for other goods and services, the objective is to identify delivery pools that incorporate the service patterns of most of an area's residents, and that allow individuals the option of several alternative choices. In practical terms, this means that the size of 'natural markets' will differ considerably for different types of health services. In particular, primary care and social service markets will tend to be considerably smaller – both geographically and demographically – than those of speciality hospital services.

A second general principle for designing competitive market units concerns the reimbursement criteria incorporated into newly flexible budgets. The central mechanism for both provider institutions and personnel salaries should combine a pre-defined 'base' level with subsequent 'adjustments' tied to various performance measures. This 'base plus adjustments' formula would be constructed of different components for institutions and personnel staff, and for the capital, primary care or social service sub-sectors of the delivery system. The objective in all instances is to mix a degree of financial certainty (the base) with a degree of financial risk (the adjustments) in a manner that can stimulate operating efficiency and responsiveness to patients without endangering the broader effectiveness-linked social objectives of the overall system.

A number of additional points can be made within the context of this broad financial framework. With regard to flexible budgeting for provider institutions – health centres, hospital clinics, nursing homes – the amount of financial transaction should be a predetermined 'internal' or 'transfer' price rather than a true cost-based price. This approach creates a system which is easy for health professionals to understand. Moreover, as the Stockholm County experiments with primary and maternity care indicate, as well as the Malmöhus model, such a transfer price based system is relatively inexpensive to administer, in apparent contrast to the buy–sell model developed by Kopparberg County. Depending upon the particular design of the public firms, the transfer price can be set somewhat lower than the average operating cost for all units, eliminating the danger of regulatory pricing that encourages 'practice to the mean', as well as encouraging most provider units to re-evaluate their cost patterns.

With regard to personnel, most particularly physicians, the financial incentives of the 'base plus adjustments' model can be intentionally designed to supplement and reinforce existing professional and peer prestige incentives. For example, as in the Finnish Personal Doctor Programme, general practitioners can receive additional compensation for what is, in effect, developing their own individual medical practice inside the walls of the health centre. As a result, GPs can obtain increased salaries for fulfilling their own professional objective of providing higher quality patient care (Vohlonen *et al.,* 1989). The ability of a properly designed planned market to integrate professional with financial incentives is essential given the central importance of professional as against financial incentives in determining physician practice patterns (Young and Saltman, 1985; Saltman, 1986).

A final point concerning budgeting for public competition is that the transition from fixed to flexible 'base plus adjustment' arrangements could be phased into operation over a period of several years. While specific approaches can vary, one logical format would be to begin with personnel salaries (to reward better performance) and then progress to institutional operating and, lastly, capital payments. Another alternative would be to start with a high fixed base and only minimal at-risk adjustments, to be followed over several budget years by step-wise increases in the at-risk component. One might precede each change with a 'shadow budget' that would enable providers to gauge the likely effect of the coming change and to adapt to the new incentives before they are actually introduced into the relevant budget. The phase-in and the shadow-budget procedures should help to reduce disruption for personnel and patients during the transition period.

ADMINISTERING FLEXIBLE BUDGETS: SOME PROPOSALS FOR IMPLEMENTATION

This section considers how the concept of flexible budgeting might be applied to annual operating budgets for general practitioners, primary care group practices and health centres, and for inpatient hospital care. Our discussion below is limited in a number of important respects. First, it is not comprehensive, in that it does not cover other categories of health institutions (rehabilitation and mental institutions, nursing homes), numerous health sector personnel (hospital specialists, nursing personnel social workers) or long-term capital budgets. Second, being segmented and sequential, this presentation format does not directly attempt to integrate performance incentives and budget allocations across the several health care sub-sectors in an appropriately coordinated manner.

Third, and perhaps most important, the managerial issues we discuss provide only one element within a well-devised management control system that is acceptable to health care professionals. While the discussion in this section focuses almost exclusively on financial incentives, the impact and suitability of salary-related increases, as already noted, is highly circumscribed by such factors as professional values and peer prestige, as well as by high marginal tax rates in Northern European countries. Too great an emphasis on financial incentives alone, focused exclusively on individuals rather than on teams, can create perverse outcomes that involve 'working' the reimbursement system. Indeed, as Swedish experience has demonstrated, relatively primitive budgeting mechanisms can be quite effective as long as they link performance to job security as well as institutional resources. Thus, it is essential to note that the explicitly managerial model developed below must be appropriately incorporated in a broadly conceived managerial framework that recognizes and responds to other key incentives that motivate professional behaviour.

Primary care physicians

There are several alternative mechanisms by which the salary structure of the general practitioner (GP) can be tied to specific performance measures. One key productivity measure, linked to the right of patients to choose (and easily change) their primary care doctor, would be the number of individuals enrolled on the GP's list (his or her 'public market share'). A second would reflect the degree to which a given GP's practice pattern coincides on certain key quality and cost measures with those of colleagues nationwide (his or her 'performance'). These two measures, when combined, would replace fixed salary structures with an integrated set of internally consistent incentives that promote simultaneously greater levels of production efficiency, health effectiveness and responsiveness to patients.

One initial prototype was the Personal Doctor Programme in Finland. As noted in Chapter 5, the salary model identified as the most effective alternative has three segments: a base component for education and experience, of roughly 20 per cent; a capitation component calculated according to the number of enrolled individuals (on an age- and sex-adjusted basis) on the GP's list, of roughly 60 per cent; and a coverage component, to encourage GPs to schedule at least one visit per year for each enrollee, of roughly 20 per cent. Although the Personal Doctor model incorporates public market share as well as a key performance indicator for preventive care, it does not evaluate a GP's curative performance (for example, on hospital referral rates). Moreover, this three-part salary model is only for primary medical services, and thus it does nor resolve difficult questions regarding the coordination of primary medical with primary health services (maternal and child health, school health, health education), or technical issues involved in linking the salaries of primary medical and primary health nurses to this new GP model (Vohlonen *et al.*, 1989).

There are a variety of key indicators for GP practice patterns which could be surrogates for improved efficiency and effectiveness of both curative and preventive care. One could, for example, adjust a GP's salary either up or down, by some factor (say 10 per cent) based upon a combination of (a) the annual referral rate to specialist care, on an age- and sex-standardized basis, and (b) the proportion of preventive activities to curative patient visits. Where organizationally and culturally appropriate, these indices could be tied to the performance of a physician group or a clinical department (Saltman, 1986), or to the mandatory introduction of a second clinical opinion for specialist referrals. The combined impact of these two readily calculated 'performance' measures, if linked to a salary model constructed upon 'public market share', would be to gear the salary-based incentives of general practitioners to more responsive, higher quality, less intensive and less wasteful primary medical as well as primary health care. Moreover, this goal could be accomplished with the same pool of salary money being expended under the present budgeting structure, by aligning the reimbursement levels for each component within the GP's salary structure, most particularly the capitation figure.

It should be noted that, in the Finnish model, the volume-related component of the physician reimbursement structure was linked to new rather than to repeat patient visits. Hence, incentives were directed towards the preventive goal of population coverage rather than towards 'turnstile' visits from the same patients. Conversely, the inclusion of a referral pattern indicator would serve, if added to the Personal Doctor approach, to discourage increased or inappropriate referrals to hospital specialists.

Overall, a redesigned GP reimbursement system may produce a greater number of total GP visits because of increased patient access to a physician they wish to see and annual visits by a higher percentage of the total population. There will probably be, on the other hand, some cost saving to the hospital sector created by a reduction in inappropriate referrals to hospital specialists. Both outcomes were observed during the 1985–7 Finnish demonstration project (Vohlonen *et al.*, 1989).

This managerial model may well be appropriate in the British as well as the Nordic context. Although British GPs, as independent entrepreneurs working under contract to the Family Health Service Authorities of the NHS, already receive a substantial segment of their earnings on a list-tied capitated basis, they have not had their income adjusted for any performance measure regarding curative care (they do receive additional payments for certain preventive services). While the issue of clinical audit of GPs has been raised periodically, there is little mention of linking GP performance on these measures to their financial return. On the contrary, discussion has focused more on establishing an accrediting process in which clinical audit would be explicitly separated from GPs' earnings schedules. Moreover, under the 1989 proposals concerning patient choice, patients will still be required to obtain the written assent of the new GP, and to have their choice approved by the Family Health Service Authority. Thus, currently proposed British reforms continue to fall short of satisfying the criteria for the managerial approach to public competition sketched out above.

Group practices and health centres

The objective of flexible budgeting for publicly administered group practices and primary health centres is to make these budgets, like the salary structure of the GP, contingent upon (a) public market share, (b) internal efficiency and (c) health-related effectiveness. Broadly speaking, there are two different types of public competition mechanisms that can be adopted in pursuit of these three objectives. One approach relies predominantly upon what could be termed 'horizontal competition', in which market design concentrates upon stimulating group practices or primary health centres to compete among themselves for patient or public market share. A second approach adds in 'vertical competition' as well, in which group practices or health centres also hold hospital budgets, and thus hospital specialists and clinics must compete among themselves for their share of GP referrals. While the first approach emphasizes competition at the primary care level, the second creates competition *between* primary and hospital levels as well as *within* each of those levels. Referring back to planned market experiments currently underway, the first approach resembles in part that pursued in the initial Stockholm experiments with patient choice, while the second, multi-level, approach has similarities with the 1989 white paper proposal for budget-holding GPs in the UK and with elements of the forthcoming Stockholm and Kopparberg experiments to base curative budgets within primary health care boards.

Whichever design is adopted, the central mechanism for establishing group practice or health centre budgets is much the same. Once overall cost data have been developed for the health services within a defined internally competitive area, the total annual value of that 'public market' becomes known. To obtain the proper budget amount for a particular group practice or health centre, one would calculate the ratio of that facility's total number of capitated patients (on an age- and sex-adjusted basis) to the total number of patients within the competitive district, create a fraction, and multiply by the total annual planned budget. This ratio could be recalculated, say monthly, with the monthly budget becoming one-twelfth of the annual amount (perhaps seasonally adjusted to reflect peaks and troughs in patient demand).

The calculation of efficiency and effectiveness measures with which to modify this basic 'public market' figure would be dependent upon which of the two types of public competition is adopted. In both instances, however, financially linked performance criteria should be consistent with the measures utilized to adjust a GP's salary, but should involve different measures so as to broaden the assessment range. In horizontal competition, if GP practice patterns are expected to reflect average annual referral patterns, then perhaps the group practice or health centre budgets might be raised or lowered depending on whether the total (age- and sex-adjusted) length of stay of its enrollees in acute hospital beds is below or above the national (or regional) average. This adjustment would reward group practices or health centres that facilitate an early return of patients to less intensive and less expensive ambulatory treatment. Similarly, if GPs' salaries reflect the ratio of preventive to curative visits, a group practice or health centre budget might be adjusted by the percentage of the total target population seen for maternal and child health. These adjustments could be as much as 3 to 5 per cent of total budget.

With the adoption of 'vertical competition', in which the competitive market also focuses on utilization rates for hospital services, performance indicators would most probably emphasize national standards for quality of care. At the primary care level, these might involve practising at or below the national average for total number of patients with preventable clinical conditions like essential hypertension or low birth weight babies. At the hospital level, as noted in the section on hospitals below, one might adopt standards regarding infection rates or re-admission rates.

Various design issues emerge when emphasis is placed upon direct financial incentives at the primary care level. One particularly complicated issue concerns the proper budget mechanism to accommodate capital depreciation (for equipment) and rent (for premises). While capital depreciation typically has not been a part of budgets in most publicly operated health systems (Saltman, 1985a, 1987; Maxwell, 1988), there is increasing interest in building it into future full-cost operating budgets in both Sweden (SIAR, 1990) and the UK (Key, 1988a; HMSO, 1989). This reflects a broader trend of following private sector accounting conventions, which can be observed in an increasing number of publicly operated health systems in Northern Europe.

For publicly operated health centres in the Nordic countries, the largest capital expense involves office and clinic space – often in the form of free-standing publicly owned buildings. Present capital-budgeting practices, which place the initial construction cost and subsequent operating expenses (heat, light, maintenance) on separate municipal or regional accounts, do not provide an appropriate costing basis for a public competition based system. In particular, if publicly operated health centres are to receive financial incentives for increased 'public market share' they (like privately operated group practices in the UK) should also have linked capital resources to facilitate expansion of available space as required by their patient levels. Equally importantly, health centres with decreasing public market share should face revenue-related pressure to reduce their physical size.

A suitable mechanism to implement capital costing for publicly operated primary care would be to establish an independent property management company to own health-related buildings, similar to the present building authority approach employed for non-health facilities in certain Swedish counties. This publicly operated company could charge rent to existing health centres, to be renegotiated as a particular health centre requires more or less space. Further, the property management agency could be empowered to lease unoccupied space to other public sector (social service, pharmacy) as well as private sector companies.

The hospital sector

The degree and type of hospital budgeting required under public competition is contingent upon which of the two options is adopted in the design of the public market for primary care services. If a horizontal competition approach is selected, then a parallel process of public market design is necessary at the hospital or hospital clinic level. Adoption of vertical competition incorporates most hospital budget issues into the financial incentives for budget-holding group practices or health centres.

In the first, separate sector approach a complicated process of restructuring hospital budgets must be undertaken. As with rate-setting efforts in pluralist delivery systems like the United States, the central design question is the composition of the competing groups. The objective should be to create competition for a functionally tied, capped budget among similar clinics across several different hospitals. This type of grouping mechanism is obviously insufficient within individual health districts for certain intensive activities, since demographic rationalities may dictate that a district should have only one facility – for orthopaedic surgery, for example. Moreover, the grouping notion is unlikely to be useful inside individual university hospitals. However, since public competition is designed to take place not only within districts but also *across* districts, with the transference of funds among districts based on services delivered, the limitations of intra-district competition at the hospital level become less of an obstacle. In this situation, the solution probably lies with regionally defined markets incorporating several separately budgeted service districts.

The process of constructing horizontal competition among 'like groups' in hospitals can sidestep certain issues that typically confront hospital budgeting efforts, including the question of specifying case-mix adjusted patient categories and, with it, the danger of distorting patient care decisions through perverse incentives for budget-maximizing behaviour. Existing annual allocations across each category of care can be totalled, divided by the expected number of cases, and assigned a 'case price', through which all provider units within that category can be compensated for their public market share. While any transfer price system needs to reflect reliable cost data, and should incorporate reasonable approximations for different levels of resource consumption for different types of patients, this type of pricing structure need not match the precise figures necessary for participation in a private sector commercial market. As a consequence, a transfer pricing system need *not* descend to the levels of administrative expense and software complexity (as well as perverse production incentives) often attributed in the United States to Medicare's diagnostic related groups (DRG) system (Sapolsky, 1987).

In a public competition approach, with its emphasis upon normative as well as economic objectives, it would be essential to adjust new price and volume data by several broadly defined production efficiency and health effectiveness criteria. A particular specialist grouping in a competitive market sub-sector might have its 'public market share' modified by whether its (adjusted) clinical treatment pattern is above or below the national average on one or two key quality indicators. Depending upon the speciality, these indicators might include a clinic's mortality rate, its infection rate and perhaps its re-admission rate. To ensure that these indicators are appropriate as well as professionally palatable, they should ideally be selected or at least ratified by the clinicians whose practice patterns they will evaluate. If the clinic budgeting process remains on a per-patient-day basis (rather than a per-case or DRG-style payment basis), an additional adjustment might be made for above or below average age-adjusted length of stay.

As the above sketch for horizontal competition in the hospital sector suggests, it is essential to design the correct mix of incentives into the budgeting structure. Among other difficulties, practical necessity may require the development of monitoring standards based upon past practice patterns, which in turn may reflect clinically inappropriate incentives generated by previous budgeting systems. While the development of new normative standards, whether through consensus conferences among medical professionals (Andreasen, 1988; Wortman *et al.*, 1988; Calltorp, 1988) or by establishing hospital-specific practice protocols (Saltman, 1986), might be conceptually preferable, this can be a tedious and even counterproductive process.[1] Moreover, the flexible budgeting module sketched out above does not include changes in salary arrangements for hospital specialists, which can raise complicated questions of fitting together incentives for inpatient ward and outpatient polyclinic practice. As noted previously, it is also important to discuss the role of prestige-tied rather than strictly financial incentives to encourage more efficient and effective physician behaviour (Young and Saltman, 1985).

FURTHER REFLECTIONS

The three applications of flexible budgeting sketched out above seek to satisfy the core requirements for public competition. The criteria they employ have been selected to be relatively easy to calculate, on readily obtainable data and in a manner that can be understood by the providers who will ultimately be judged by them. As such, these applications reflect two central tenets of good management control theory: they are controllable by those whom they hold accountable, and they provide a 'good' outcome for the organization as a whole when they provide a 'good' outcome for the individual provider or provider institution (Young and Saltman, 1985).

One of the central challenges of public competition is to link

newly flexible budgets both horizontally, to out-of-district providers and institutions, and, most importantly, vertically across the
separate hospital, primary care and social service sub-sectors within
each flexible budget 'district'. Experiments with vertical competition in Sweden and, potentially, the United Kingdom will
attempt to forge these linkages between primary medical and
hospital care. A similar across-sector arrangement is conceivable
with social services, giving primary health centres control over the
health-related segments of the social services budget. However, the
necessary cross-jurisdictional re-alignment of budgetary responsibility (from local municipality to district or county) would in most
instances complicate such a process. One interesting experiment in
1988 in Denmark might be adapted for use with a public competition approach. In North Jutland, the municipally operated
social services were given five days to 'take back' a patient once the
hospital clinic notified social services that an inpatient was ready for
discharge. If the social service sector was not able to place the
patient properly within that period, then social services had to pay
the hospital for each subsequent day of care (K. Christensen,
personal communication).

It should be emphasized that, in flexible budgeting as elsewhere,
public competition is a broad zone of activity rather than a precise
recipe for organizational reconfiguration. The specific character of
flexible budgeting can be adjusted to meet a wide variety of criteria,
including the availability of adequate information and the normative objectives of the system's publicly elected overseers. Indeed,
precisely this dynamic character is an important strength of the
public competition approach.

THE BROADER PERSPECTIVE

The central objective of public competition is to create an efficient
public market for health care services. In this context, efficiency has
a considerably broader meaning than that typically assigned to it
within neo-classical economics. First, public competition would be
economically efficient at both the individual institutional and the
system levels, in that it would require providers and provider
institutions to compete for public market share, both for personal
remuneration and for long-term institutional survival. Second,
public competition would be personally efficient at the patient level,

in that it would meet 'individual wants' – or patient preferences – through the combined mechanisms of patient choice of physician and institutions, and national monitoring of quality standards. Third, public competition would be politically efficient at the governmental level, in that it would maintain continued accountability for demographically and epidemiologically defined 'public needs', as well as normative objectives concerning equity and access to a universal system of quality care.

From a managerial perspective, public competition has the advantage of being readily understandable both by the administrative and planning personnel who must design new systems and by health providers who will be judged by their performance within it. Conceptually speaking it is a 'simple system', in which organizational goals are clearly communicated.

Public competition is also a model of organizational decentralization which opens up new possibilities for worker participation in policy and administrative aspects of institutional decision-making. Moving beyond concepts of consensus management and codetermination generally, public competition creates the option to integrate institutional personnel within an interactive decision-making process vital to sustaining the provider institution's future. Since, under flexible budgeting, the patient's assessment of the quality of services becomes an essential measurement of performance, a health centre or department clinic will feel considerable financial pressure to reorganize on an interactive basis in order to satisfy patient expectations. Similarly, personnel within each health centre or hospital 'public firm' will probably want to participate in setting the two or three quality-tied performance measures upon which their institutional budgets and salaries will be adjusted.

The crux of the public competition approach is the relatively unrestricted choice within the public system of where and by whom health care is delivered. The administration of health services is placed in a subordinate role to patient care decisions, and political bodies will no longer be entitled to micro-manage institutional-level behaviour. Indeed, the role of the public owning agency becomes one of supporting patients' delivery decisions with appropriate shifts in health service resources between facilities as well as with enhanced incentives for efficiency within each delivery unit. The central driving force of public competition, therefore, relies in practice upon what neo-classical economists insist in theory is the central decision-making factor in a market-based system: individual choice.

Public competition, however, introduces patient choice within a wholly public health delivery system. Although providers and delivery institutions have professional and financial incentives to satisfy individual wants, providers' success in doing so will be unrelated to the usual exchange value consequences concerning profit and capital accumulation. Moreover, precisely because it remains a public system, it will not be possible for providers to concentrate solely on individual wants to the exclusion of public needs. That is, the health delivery system will remain structured in terms of value-in-use to the patient, and can continue to provide preventive and curative care for all, including the less well off, the elderly, the chronically ill and other high-consumption patient groupings.

Public competition is intended to retain two central features of existing publicly operated health systems. First, health care budgets would remain global and prospective, with total expenditure for each delivery sub-sector set in advance. In their competition for public market share, health providers could only seek a larger share of what would remain a fixed resource allocation. There is, consequently, little danger of creating open-ended expenditures, a standard difficulty with pluralist and private delivery systems. Second, national standards of care and quality control could be created under the supervision of a national monitoring agency. The Swedish approach of compiling key statistics for publication could be enhanced to prevent unwarranted variations in the volume or quality of care delivered.

Beyond these two points, several additional issues concerning the implementation of public competition deserve brief attention. Perhaps the most important is that a public competition approach need not create major new administrative costs (as clearly indicated by Swedish experience). For primary care, patient choice of site and provider could be administered through a regular open enrolment period each year. The British and Danish experiences with general practitioner lists (as well as the Finnish Personal Doctor experiment) confirm that this system need not entail large expenditures of administrative time or funds.

For hospital care, a reimbursement mechanism for compensating a hospital which treats a patient from another budgeting district already exists in many systems. The introduction of public competition might entail certain modifications in existing arrangements:

it might be necessary, for example, to review current *per diem* reimbursement structures to prevent unintended inter-district subsidies. Certainly, it will be necessary to re-invigorate existing payment mechanisms to make them contemporaneous with out-of-district service delivery.

A further administrative saving from a properly articulated public competition model would reflect its ability to reduce high insurance costs for employed individuals who must wait in queues for elective specialist treatment. Under a public competition approach, no formal arrangement with publicly operated providers would be necessary to speed employed patients through the queues. Rather, the national insurance system would only need to stipulate that employed patients are obligated to seek out an appropriate treatment provider with a relatively short waiting period.

A related administrative issue concerns the usefulness of public competition as a framework for pursuing a locally controlled, primary care based health strategy. As noted above, public competition is fully consistent with local control, whether at district, sub-district, municipal, or sub-municipal level, since the competing public firms remain entirely within the public sector. Indeed, local control suggests that many aspects of individual wants will be implemented rapidly by local group practices or health centres, minimizing the likelihood that individuals would choose to receive their care at a more distant facility. Local control also suggests the likelihood of close monitoring of local service standards and patient volume, since falling patient loads (assuming static area population) could lead to reduced resource allocation in the budgeting cycle. Further, if cut-backs are indicated, locally controlled primary care units are least likely to compound their problems by inadvertently cutting the most essential local services. Local control thus increases flexibility in adjusting patterns of service delivery to changing levels of resources.

It should be noted that the behavioural and financial incentives established, and the data-collection system as well, could be structured along substantive professional as well as financial lines. For example, a primary care reimbursement system could reward physician behaviour that emphasizes certain types of preventive screenings. In this fashion, normative policy as well as financial efficiency concerns could be incorporated into the new model's incentive structure. The inclusion of both policy and financial goals in the incentive system also accommodates the practical reality that, at the point of clinical delivery, physicians exercise *de facto* power over a considerable segment of the health sector's resource allocation process (Saltman, 1985b).

Finally, public competition requires substantial flexibility from health sector labour unions and, in systems with elected local health officials, from politicians. Support from labour unions is essential given that a high percentage of employees are organized in most Northern European health systems. The unions, in particular, need to endorse flexibility in the assignment of employee worksites and, like their private sector counterparts, accept employee bonus schemes and other direct and indirect economic incentives to stimulate productivity and effectiveness.

In the Nordic countries, local health politicians must accept a shift in their role. The traditional planning-oriented delivery structure encouraged regional or municipal politicians to focus predominantly on supply-side issues: obtaining additional resources, maintaining employment levels, building new capital facilities and allocating the annual budget. In a public competition approach, health politicians as well as health planners will be forced to adjust this provider orientation to fit demand-side, patient-generated concerns. Health sector officials will need to view themselves not as the ultimate arbiters of health resource allocation, but rather as the architects of broad institutional arrangements within which effective public competition can occur. The specific responsibility of the health politician will thus be to facilitate the smooth running of a carefully constructed marketplace within which patients choose from a variety of high quality public providers, while at the same time ensuring that the new system continues to satisfy public needs as well as patient demands.

NOTE

1 An example of the latter are some of the Swedish medical care programmes (Vårdprogram), which seek to integrate treatment across multiple sites for certain common conditions (breast cancer, hypertension, lower back pain, etc.) (Pine *et al.,* 1988). However, some county councils have felt that the treatment patterns recommended were too expensive, and hence they have not elected to implement them.

10

PLANNED MARKETS IN POLITICAL PERSPECTIVE

Current experiments with planned market models represent an important step towards major structural reform within publicly operated health systems in Northern Europe. Seeking to escape inappropriate policy paradigms and anachronistic organizational patterns, health sector professionals, managers and politicians have embarked upon a collective search for alternative models of service design and delivery. While some experiments raise sensitive issues about the appropriate mission of publicly operated systems, the majority of these planned market efforts seek mechanisms which will reinforce the core values that publicly operated health systems have traditionally embodied.

The central question posed by this swirl of activities is whether radical, although often partial, experiments in the present period will lead to instrumental and ultimately strategic processes of change in the foreseeable future. It is this transformation – from issue-driven pragmatic reform to conceptually coherent strategic reform – that will guarantee the long-term future of publicly operated systems. Further, as demonstrated by the considerable differences in planned market mechanisms currently under consideration, not every attempt at strategic reform views this future through the same conceptual lens. The key question thus becomes not only whether a transition to strategic reform will occur but also which strategic reform model strikes the optimal balance between security and challenge in the organization of publicly operated health systems generally.

Our analysis of the appropriate role for markets in health care begins from the observation that every market is, by definition as well as in practice, a political market. Once a policy-maker moves beyond the myths and symbols with which neo-classical economics wraps itself, he or she directly confronts highly political design questions focused on who gets what, when and how – questions that Harold Lasswell argued to be the *sine qua non* of politics (Lasswell, 1936). As we noted in the Preface, these market design questions involve a series of critical choices. In which sub-sectors of the health system will competition be introduced? Will incentives be structured on cost, on quality or on market share? Which actors (physicians, managers, patients) will be the focus of these incentives? Who will be accountable for capital allocation and by what means? Who will maintain standards for quality and access and by what means? How will market style incentives be adapted for use within 'natural monopolies' in the health sector? How will 'regulatory capture' by either public or private enterprises be forestalled? How will a market-generated explosion of new administrative costs be prevented? In which activities will integration and cooperation be fostered instead of competition?

In pursuing answers to these design questions, political decision-makers take on the responsibilities of what economists call the 'market-maker' – that is, the trader who puts buyer and seller together to create a market. In a planned market, it is the political decision-makers who directly construct the organizational framework within which competitive behaviour occurs, and they are responsible for making whatever structural adaptations might be necessary to ensure that the market does not break down. The clearest confirmation of this market-maker role can be seen in the rubber windmill experiment in May 1990 in the United Kingdom, in which national policy-makers sought to learn more about the key structural elements necessary to keep their particular planned market model running smoothly.

The political character of the market design process can also be observed in the emerging role of public firms within these new planned markets. In all three country studies, the characteristics of the public firms under consideration will be subject to strict political accountability for their market-driven behaviour. Even in the UK, where the mixed market character of the proposal required the greatest degree of independence for public firms (as self-governing trusts), the 1989 white paper explicitly gave broad reserve powers to ministers to intervene if the new markets' outcome became politically undesirable (HMSO, 1989). In practice, key economic questions such as market contestability and bankruptcy would, in the British, Swedish and Finnish contexts alike, become directly political questions, to be decided by the politically responsible officials in consultation with their policy support staff. As a consequence, while public firms could be expected to take consider-able advantage of their new status to pursue a wide variety of internal efficiencies, these public firms would be required to rein in their behaviour should it threaten the political or normative objectives they were initially established to achieve.

A planned market might not allow total decision-making auton-omy for the firms within it, but this is not entirely different from present reality within many private sectors of the economy. Quite contrary to assumptions in economists' models about perfect markets and perfect competition, with a dominant role for the 'invisible hand', firms in many industries operate according to what Arthur Okun, a former Chairman of the President's Council of Economic Advisors in the United States, labelled the 'invisible handshake' (Okun, 1981). By this, Okun means that routine and automatic price arrangements are often agreed upon in order to create continuity and convenience of supply. One result of this market cooperation is that prices become 'sticky' and do not directly reflect shifts in market conditions. Thus, although planned markets clearly differ in the purpose, identity and perhaps scope of the market limitations generated, the existence of these limitations need not undercut desirable market-oriented behaviour in public any more than it does in many private firms.

These various design issues all strongly suggest that, in the adaptation of market mechanisms to publicly operated health sys-tems, key economic questions become directly subordinated to the political or normative objectives of the political decision-makers who construct planned markets, and who will be held publicly accountable for their performance. This assessment stands in direct opposition to the claims of the so-called 'public choice' school of economists, who argue that elected officials and civil servants primarily act as self-maximizing rational economic creatures (Downs, 1957; Buchanan and Tullock, 1962; Buchanan, 1969). Rather, in the planned market debate currently underway inside publicly operated health systems, neo-classical economic argu-ments are being treated as simply one among many different types of political argument – and not the most persuasive one at that.

Seen historically, this emphasis on the political purposes of economic markets returns to the original understanding of Adam

Smith and his Scottish forebear, Robert Hutchinson. In Smith's view, markets existed within a broad social and moral context which structured private as well as public life. Market activity was a mechanism to achieve economic efficiencies *inside* a moral community, not in opposition to that community. Thus, individual pursuit of self-interest was seen to be in the service of, rather than the replacement for, social and moral objectives in the community interest. In this respect, one can argue that public firms, if designed to reinforce (rather than undermine) collective community objectives, can generate much the same socially appropriate forms of economic behaviour that Smith originally envisioned for entrepreneurial individuals.

In our discussion of planned market models, we have argued that the normative and political implications of strategic reform models should be viewed as being as important as their economic consequences. Our concerns about the counterproductive dynamics triggered off by various privatized and mixed market models of health care reform strongly reflect this central conceptual perspective. We should also cite the dismal experience of the United States, with its particular version of price-based competition among for-profit private firms, as an example of an approach to health care reform which public health systems should avoid.

Of the various planned market models proposed or discussed, we continue to believe that a public competition approach remains best suited to achieving a satisfactory mix of normative and political as well as economic objectives. As we conceive it, public competition partially uncouples health sector management from political control on matters of economic productivity, but retains public responsibility for normative outcomes through its social definition of the efficiencies to be achieved. Properly constructed, public competition would trigger a process of strategic reform based upon 'creative restruction' rather than Schumpeterian 'creative destruction'. The dynamic of change, while nearly as thoroughgoing as Schumpeter's, would minimize social as well as economic costs of change which, in a publicly operated system, are borne by the same publicly responsible and publicly financed entity. This capacity to minimize social costs in the use of market mechanisms is of particular importance in periods of broad economic recession, when the combination of reduced public sector revenues and increased unemployment could rapidly destabilize less publicly accountable forms of planned markets.

The most crucial characteristic of public competition is its ability to confer real practical power upon the patient. By linking patient choice of public provider with the distribution of institutional revenues and personnel incomes in a defined public market, public competition can transform the patient from the object into the subject of the health care system. Unlike competitive mechanisms in the United States like health maintenance organizations (HMO) and preferred provider organizations (PPO), which severely restrict patient choice in pursuit of cost efficiencies, unlike the manager-led form of mixed competition proposed for the United Kingdom in the 1989 white paper, which would further restrict the already limited influence of patients over where and from whom they receive care, in a public competition approach the patient's decision about where to obtain care becomes the decisive factor for steering system-wide resource flows. As a direct result of its patient-driven character, unlike in private sector competition models, public competition can achieve cost efficiencies without risking substantial reductions in either the quality of curative care on the one hand, or the provision of primary and preventive services on the other.

Finally, as we contend with our argument about voice and choice, public competition's emphasis on empowering patients enhances the democratic character of both health care system and society overall. Quite opposite to the atomized notion of empowerment popular in conservative circles in the United States, which relies upon a Lockean 'freedom-from' using fixed price vouchers for privately provided services, public competition pursues individual choice as part of a broader strategy of 'freedom-through' collective political accountability. By conjoining process democracy to content democracy – by recognizing the value of civil democracy in the provision of public sector human services generally – public competition can help to re-legitimize publicly operated health systems in the eyes of the citizens they serve. In the final analysis, beyond questions of cost efficiencies or quality of care or professional job satisfaction, this may well prove to be the strongest recommendation for adopting a public competition approach.

The development of this process of strategic reform will be influenced by a variety of factors. The continuing process of economic globalization can be expected to maintain pressures within countries in Northern Europe to increase exports, expand productivity and reduce costs in private industry. To the extent that health care expenditure along with other components of the social wage are viewed as consumption, increased global economic competitiveness can influence the type of strategic reform model adopted – an argument made with regard to the 1989 white paper proposals in the United Kingdom (Warner, 1989). Similar pressures may well ensue in the wake of the 1992 removal of restraints to trade within the European Community – not only for the 12 EC countries but also for their EFTA trading partners and, possibly, future members. The 1992 reform could have an impact on the health sector directly, for example by altering the labour market pool for trained medical professionals or by generating opportunities for cross-national and trans-national production of clinical services. The latter issue could become particularly important for countries which adopt a mixed public and private form of planned market, in that the European Commission's contracting requirements could force health authorities to adopt a more comprehensive and expensive bidding process. Other uncertainties are created by an ongoing process of feminization of the physician workforce, particularly within the Nordic countries, and the decreasing ratio of working age to retirement age people. Finally, the future of publicly operated health systems is necessarily linked to the future of other publicly produced human services like education and child care, and thus to long-term reform of the welfare state as a whole.

Despite the impact of these and other external changes, efforts to create and implement new planned market projects are likely to increase significantly over the decade of the 1990s. Although specific experiments will be deemed unsuccessful, and the transition from reformist to strategic reform models may develop unevenly, the underlying process of constructing consciously designed markets and firms in pursuit of public sector objectives in health policy will become increasingly attractive to health sector officials concerned with quality and equality. In the search for a new health policy paradigm for publicly operated health systems, planned markets have the capacity to integrate neo-classical economic and traditional planning approaches into a new synthesis – into a normatively as well as economically bounded health care paradigm. How this process of paradigm construction will play out is far from settled. That a new policy paradigm will in fact be produced, that this paradigm will have broadly planned market characteristics, and that it will generate major structural change throughout publicly operated health systems, now appears to be all but inevitable.

BIBLIOGRAPHY

Andersson, N. R. *et al.* (1976). *Kan Sverige styras kooperativt?* Stockholm, Tidens förlag.

Andreasen, P. B. (1988). 'Consensus conferences in different countries: aims and perspectives', *International Journal of Technology Assessment*, **4**, 395–408.

Aoki, M., Gustavsson, B. and Williamson, O. E. (eds) (1989). *The Firm as a Nexus of Treaties*. London, Sage.

Ascher, K. (1987). *The Politics of Privatization. Contracting Out Public Services*. London, Macmillan Education.

Barry, B. (1974). 'Exit, voice, and loyality: a review article', *British Journal of Political Science*, **4**, 79–107.

Berlin, I. (1969). *Four Essays on Liberty*. Oxford, Clarendon Press.

Berwick, D. M., Godfrey, A. B. and Roessner, J. (1990). *Curing Health Care: New Strategies for Quality Improvement*. San Francisco, CA., Jossey-Bass.

Bevan, G. (1988). How should district allocations be altered for changes in cross boundary flows?', *British Medical Journal*, **296**, 144–5.

Bevan, G. (1989). 'Reforming UK health care: internal markets or emergent planning?', *Fiscal Studies*, **10**, 53–71.

Bevan, G. and Marinker, M. (1989). *Greening the White Paper: a Strategy for NHS Reform*. London, The Social Market Foundation.

Birch, A. H. (1975). 'Economic models in political science: the case of exit, voice, and loyalty', *British Journal of Political Science*, **5**, 65–82.

Birch, S. and Maynard, A. (1988). 'Performance indicators', in R. J. Maxwell (ed.) *Reshaping the Natural Health Service*. London, Policy Journals, pp. 51–64.

Borgonovi, E. (1990). 'Competition in the public healthcare system: a reference framework', in *Proceedings of the Conference on Paradoxes of Competition*, Nuffield Institute, University of Leeds.

Bosworth, B. and Rivlin, A. (eds) (1987). *The Swedish Economy*. Washington, DC, Brookings Institution.

Brazier, J. (1987). 'Accounting for cross boundary flows', *British Medical Journal*, **295**, 898–900.

Buchanan, J. M. (1969). *Cost and Choice: an Inquiry in Economic Theory*. Chicago, Markham.

Buchanan, J. and Tullock, G. (1962). *The Calculus of Consent. Logical Foundations of Constitutional Democracy*. Ann Arbor, University of Michigan Press.

Butler, E. and Pirie, M. (1988). *Health Management Units: the Operation of an Internal Market within a National Health Service*. London, Adam Smith Institute.

Calltorp, J. (1988). 'Consensus development conferences in Sweden: effects on health policy and administration', *International Journal of Technology Assessment in Health Care*, **4**(1), 75–88.

Cassirer, E. (1954). *The Question of Jean-Jacques Rousseau*. New York, Columbia University Press.

Castles, F. G. (1978). *The Social Democratic Image of Society: a Study of the Achievements and Origins of Scandinavian, Social Democracy in Comparative Perspective*. London, Routledge and Kegan Paul.

Christianson, J. B. and Hillman, D. G. (1986). *Health Care for Indigent and Competitive Contracts: the Arizona Experiment*. Ann Arbor, MI, Health Administration Press.

Chubb, J. E. and Moe, T. M. (1990). *Politics, Markets and America's Schools*. Washington, DC, Brookings Institution.

Cole, G. D. H. (1920). *Guild Socialism Re-stated*. London, Leonard Parsons.

Coles, J. (1988). 'Clinical budgeting as a management tool', in R. Maxwell (ed.) *Reshaping the National Health Service*. London, Policy Journals, pp. 126–37.

Crozier, M. (1964). *The Bureaucratic Phenomenon*. Chicago, University of Chicago Press.

Culyer, A. J. and Jönsson, B. (eds) (1986). *Public and Private Health Services*. Oxford, Basil Blackwell.

de Faramond, G., Harrington, M. and Martin, A. (1982). 'Sweden seen from the outside', in B. Rydén and V. Bergström, (eds) *Sweden: Choices for Economic and Social Policy in the 1980s*. London, George Allen & Unwin.

D'Onofrio, C. and Muller, P. (1977). 'Consumer problems with prepaid health plans in California', *Public Health Reports*, **92**, 121–34.

Downs, A. (1957). *An Economic Theory of Democracy*. New York, Harper.

Drummond, M. and Maynard, A. (1988). 'Efficiency in the National Health Service: lessons from abroad', *Health Policy*, **9**, 59–74.

Eklund, L. K. and Kronvall, K. F. (1988). 'Responsiveness, decentralization and implications for the roles of the employees', paper for the OECD/IULA Workshop on Urban Services and Consumer Needs,

Amsterdam, 22–25 April. Stockholm, Swedish Centre for Working Life.

Enthoven, A. (1980). *Health Plan: the Only Practical Solution to the Soaring Cost of Medical Care*. Reading, MA, Addison-Wesley.

Enthoven, A. (1985). *Reflections on the Management of the National Health Service*. London, Nuffield Provincial Hospitals' Trust.

Enthoven, A. (1986). 'Managed competition in health care and the unfinished agenda', *Health Care Financing Review*, annual supplement, 105–19.

Enthoven, A. (1991). 'Quality and health care', paper presented to a seminar at the Institute for Public Policy Research, London.

Enthoven, A. and Kronick, R. (1989). 'A consumer choice health plan for the 1990s', *New England Journal of Medicine*, **320**, 29–37; 94–101.

Erikson, R. and Åberg, R. (eds) (1987). *Welfare in Transition. A Survey of Living Conditions in Sweden 1968–81*. Oxford, Clarendon Press.

Etzioni, A. (1988). *The Moral Dimension: Toward a New Economics*. New York, Free Press.

Evans, R. (1986). 'Finding the levers, finding the courage: lessons from cost containment in North America', *Journal of Health Politics, Policy and Law*, **11**, 585–615.

Fattore, G. and Garattini, L. (1989). 'L'allocazione delle resorse finanziarie nel servizio sanitario nazionale: il quadro teorico e una soluzione practica'. *Economica Publica*, **11**, 541–56.

Finansdepartmentet (1985). *Produktions-, kostnads- och produktivitetsutveckling inom offentlig bedriven hälso- och sjukvård 1960–1980*. Stockholm, DsFi.

Finansdepartmentet (1987). *Integrering av sjukvård och sjukförsäkring*. Stockholm, DsFi.

Finnish Ministry of Social Affairs and Health (1987) *Health for All by the Year 2000: the Finnish National Health Strategy*. Helsinki, Ministry of Social Affairs and Health.

Finsinger, J., Kraft, K. and Pauly, M. (1986). 'Some observations on greater competition in the West German health-insurance system from a U.S. perspective', *Managerial and Decision Economics*, **7**, 157–61.

Flora, P. (1986–7). *Growth to Limits. The West European Welfare States Since World War II, 1–3*. Berlin and New York, Walter de Gruyter.

Framtidsgruppen (1989). *90-tals Programmet*. Stockholm, Socialdemokratiska partiet.

Freeland, M. S. *et al.* (1987). 'Selective contracting for hospital care based on volume, quality, and price: prospects, problems and unanswered questions', *Journal of Health Politics, Policy and Law*, **12**, 409–26.

Friedman, M. (1962). *Capitalism and Freedom*. Chicago, University of Chicago Press.

Friedman, M. and Friedman, R. (1981). *Free to Choose*. New York, Harcourt Brace, Jovanovich.

Gardell, B. and Gustafsson, R. Å. (1979). *Sjukvård på löpande band, Rapport från ett forskningsprojekt om sjukhusens vård och organisation.* Stockholm, Prisma.

Goldsmith, M. and Willetts, D. (1988). *Managed Health Care: a New System for a Better Health Service.* London, Centre for Policy Studies.

Golinowska, S., Tymowska, K. and Wlodarczyk, C. (1989). *In the Interest of Health of the Society: a Proposal of Health Care System Reorganization.* Warsaw, Ministry of Health.

Gorz, A. (1964). *A Strategy for Labor.* Boston, Beacon Press.

Gough, R. (1987). *Hemhjälp till Gamla.* Stockholm, Arbetslivscentrum.

Granqvist, R. (1987). *Privata och kollektiva val. En kritisk analys av Public choice-skolan.* Lund, Arkiv.

Gray, B. (ed) (1986). *For-Profit Enterprise in Health Care.* Washington, DC, Institute of Medicine.

Green, D., Neuberger, J. *et al.* (1990). *The NHS Reforms: Whatever Happened to Consumer Choice?*, Health Series No. 11. London, Institute for Economic Affairs.

Greenberg, W. (ed) (1978). *Competition in the Health Care Sector: Past, Present and Future.* Germantown, MD, Aspen System.

Gulick, L. (1937) 'Notes on the theory of organization', in L. Gulick and L. Urwick (eds) *Papers on the Science of Administration.* New York, Institute of Public Administration, pp. 3–13.

Gustavsen, B. (1990). *Dialogues and Development. Theory of Communication, Action Research and the Restructuring of Working Life* (unpublished manuscript). Stockholm, Arbetslivscentrum.

Habermas, J. (1981). *Theorie des kommunikativen Handelns.* Frankfurt Suhrkamp.

Ham, C. (1988). 'Governing the health sector: power and policy making in the English and Swedish health services', *Milbank Memorial Fund Quarterly*, **66**, 389–414.

Ham, C. and Hunter, D. J. (1988). *Managing Clinical Activity in the NHS.* London, King's Fund Institute.

Ham, C., Robinson, R. and Benzeval, M. (1990). *Health Check: Health Policy in an International Perspective.* London, King's Fund Institute.

Harrison, S. (1988a). 'The workplace and the new managerialism', in R. Maxwell (ed.) *Reshaping the National Health Service.* London, Policy Journals, pp. 141–52.

Harrison, S. (1988b). 'Health care in Britain', in R. B. Saltman (ed.) *The International Handbook of Health-Care Systems.* Westport, CT and London, Greenwood Press.

Harrison, S., Hunter, D. J., Johnston, I. and Wistow, G. (1989a). *Competing for Health: a Commentary on the NHS Review.* Leeds, Nuffield Institute.

Harrison, S., Hunter, D. J., Marnoch, G. and Pollitt, C. (1989b).

General Management in the National Health Service: Before and After the White Paper. Leeds, Nuffield Institute.

Heclo, H. and Madsen, H. (1987). *Policy and Politics in Sweden: Principled Pragmatism*. Philadelphia, PA, Temple University Press.

Heidenheimer, A. J. and Johansen, L. N. (1985). 'Organized medicine and Scandinavian professional unionism: Hospital policies and exit options in Denmark and Sweden', *Journal of Health Politics, Policy and Law*, **10**, 347–71.

Heister, P. and Gustavsson, E. (1989). 'Landstingens planerade elände', *Svenska Dagbladet*, 21 July.

Hertzlinger, R. and Krasker, W. S. (1987). 'Who profits from non-profits?', *Harvard Business Review*, **65**, 93–106.

Higgins, J. (1988). *The Business of Medicine: Private Health Care in Britain*. London, Macmillan Education.

Himmelstein, D. U. and Woolhandler, S. (1986). 'Cost without benefit: administrative waste in US health care', *New England Journal of Medicine*, **314**, 441–5.

Himmelstein, D. U. *et al.* (1989). 'A national health program for the United States', *New England Journal of Medicine*, **320**, 102–8.

Hirschman, A. (1970). *Exit, Voice, and Loyalty*. Cambridge, MA, Harvard University Press.

HMSO (1988). *Community Care: Agenda for Action* (Griffiths Report). London, Her Majesty's Stationery Office.

HMSO (1989). *Working for Patients*. London, Her Majesty's Stationery Office.

Hood, C. (1988). 'Para-government organization in the United Kingdom', in C. Hood and G. F. Schuppert (eds) *Delivering Public Services in Western Europe: Sharing Western European Experience of Para-Government Organization*. London, Sage Publications, pp. 75–93.

Håkansson, S., Paulson, E. and Kogeus, K. (1988). 'Prospects for using DRGs in Swedish Hospitals', *Health Policy*, **9**, 177–92.

Institute for Health Service Management (1988). *Working Party on Alternative Delivery and Funding of Health Services: Final Report*. London, IHSM.

Jávor, A. (1990). 'The new national health fund and the health care reform in Hungary', paper presented to the WHO Meeting on New Approachs to Managing Health Services, Nuffield Institute, University of Leeds.

Jonsson, E. and Skalin, D. (eds) (1985). *Privat och offentlig sjukvård: Samverkan eller konkurrens*? Stockholm, Spri.

Kalimo, E. (1990) 'The Finnish experience', paper presented on the WHO European Region Meeting on Financing of Health Services, Copenhagen, 18–19 June.

Karolinska Hospital (1990). *Statistik från bokningsenheten, January–June 1990*. Stockholm, Kvinnokliniken (mimeo).

Kavanagh, D. (1972). 'Political behaviour and political participation', in

G. Parry (ed.) *Participation in Politics*. Manchester, Manchester University Press, pp. 103–23.

Key, T. (1988a). 'Managing the capital program', in R. Maxwell (ed.) *Reshaping the National Health Service*. London, Policy Journals, pp. 97–113.

Key, T. (1988b) 'Contracting out ancillary services', in R. Maxwell (ed.) *Reshaping the National Health Service*. London, Policy Journals, pp. 65–81.

Klein, R. (1983). *The Politics of the National Health Service*. Harlow, Longman.

Korpi, W. (1978). *The Working Class in Welfare Capitalism: Work, Unions, and Politics in Sweden*. London, Routledge and Kegan Paul.

Korpi, W. (1989). 'Power, politics and state autonomy in the development of social citizenship: social rights during sickness in eighteen OECD countries since 1930', *American Sociological Review*, **54**(3), 309–28.

Kuhn, T. S. (1962). *The Structure of Scientific Revolutions*. Chicago, University of Chicago Press.

Landstingsförbundet (1986). *Landstinget som politisk drivkraft för länets utveckling*. Stockholm, Landstingsförbundet.

Landstingsförbundet (1989). *Landstingsförbundets sammandrag av äldredelegationens förslag*. Stockholm, Landstingsförbundet.

Landstingsförbundet (1991). *Vägval: Hälso- och sjukvårdens övergripande strukturer och framtiden*. Stockholm, Landstingsförbundet.

Lapré, R. (1988). 'A new direction for the Dutch health system?', *Health Policy*, **10**, 21–32.

Lasswell, H. (1936). *Politics. Who gets What, When, How*. London, McGraw-Hill.

Launois, R., Majnoni, Stéfan, J., d'Intignano, B. and Rodwin, V. (1985). 'Les réseaux de soins coordonnés (RSC): propositions pour une réforme profonde du systéme de santé. *Revue Française des Affaires Sociales*, **1**, 37–61.

Lawrence, P. and Lorsch, J. (1967). *Organization and Environment*. Boston, Graduate School of Business Administration, Harvard University.

Leichter, H. (1979). *Comparative Health Policy*. Cambridge, Cambridge University Press.

Leijon, A.-G. and Eklund, K. (1989). Större utrymme för individen. *Dagens Nyheter*, 19 August.

Lipsky, M. (1980). *Street-Level Bureaucracy*. New York, Russel Sage Foundation.

Lively, J. (1975). *Democracy*. Oxford, Basil Blackwell.

Long, N. (1949). 'Power and administration', *Public Administration Review*, **9**, 257–69.

Lundberg, E. (1985). 'The rise and fall of the Swedish model', *Journal of Economic Literature*, **23**, 1–36.

Lynch, M. (1983). *Det Brustna Hjärtat*. Stockholm, Natur och Kultur.
McCombs, J. S. and Christenson, J. B. (1987). 'Applying competitive bidding to health care', *Journal of Health Politics, Policy and Law*, **12**, 703–22.
MacGregor, D. (1960). *The Human Side of Enterprise*. New York, McGraw-Hill.
McLachlan, G. and Maynard, A. (eds) (1982). *The Public–Private Mix for Health*. London, Nuffield Provincial Hospital Trust.
March, J. and Olsen, J. (1976). *Ambiguity and Choice in Organizations*. Oslo, Universitetsforlaget.
Maslow, A. H. (1943). 'A theory of human motivation', *Psychological Review*, **50**, 370–96.
Maxwell, R. (ed) (1988). *Reshaping the National Health Service*. London, Policy Journals.
Maynard, A. and Williams, A. (1984). 'Privatization and the National Health Service', In J. Le Grand and R. Robinson (eds) *Privatization and the Welfare State*. London, George Allen & Unwin, pp. 95–110.
Meldegaard, K. and Rold Andersen, B. (1985). *Mere liv på plejehjemmene*. Copenhagen, AKF.
Mill, J. S. (1861). *Representative Government*. Reprinted in *Utilitarianism, Liberty and Representative Government* (1944). London, Everyman, p. 193.
Miller, T. (1988). *Consulting Citizens in Sweden: Planning Participation in Context*. Stockholm, Swedish Council for Building Research, D10.
Mishra, R. (1984). *The Welfare State in Crisis*. Brighton, Wheatsheaf.
Mueller, D. C. (1979). *Public Choice*. Cambridge, Cambridge University Press.
Neuhauser, D. (1986). 'A matrix model for hospitals', in A. Kovner and D. Neuhauser (eds) *Health Services Management*, 3rd edn. Ann Arbor, MI, Health Administration Press.
Nicholl, J. P. *et al.* (1984). 'Contributions of the private sector to elective surgery in England and Wales', *Lancet*, **14**, 89–92.
Normann, R. (1986). *Service Management: Strategy and Leadership in Service Business*. Chichester, Wiley.
OECD (1987). *Administration as Service: the Public as Client*. Paris, OECD.
OECD (1992). *The Reform of Health Care: A Comparative Analysis of Seven OECD Countries*. Paris, OECD.
Öhrming, J. (1990). *Kvartersakuten: Ny Organisation och ändrat Arbetssatt inom Primarvärden*. Stockholm, Arbetslivscentrum.
Okun, A. (1981). *Prices and Quantities: a Macroeconomic Analysis*. Washington, DC, Brookings Institution.
Osborne, D. and Gaebler, T. (1991). *Reinventing Government*. Boston, Harvard Business School Press.
Parston, G. (1988). 'General management', in R. Maxwell (ed.) *Reshaping the National Health Service*. London, Policy Journals, pp. 17–33.

Pekurinen, M., Vohlonen, I. and Aro, S. (1987). *Method for Estimating the Regional Need for Health Care Resources.* Helsinki, National Board of Health in Finland.

Perrow, C. (1978). 'Demystifying organizations', in R. C. Sarri and Y. Hasenfeld (eds) *The Management of Human Services.* New York, Columbia University Press, pp. 105–20.

Petersson, O. *et al.* (1989). *Medborgarnas Makt.* Helsingborg, Carlssons bokförlag.

Pine, L., Rosenqvist, U., Rosenthal, M. and Shapiro, F. (1988). 'The Swedish medical care programs: an interim assessment', *Health Policy*, **10**, 155–76.

Piri, P. and Vohlonen, I. (1987). 'Job satisfaction among primary care personnel'. *Finnish Journal of Social Medicine*, **24**, 287–96 (in Finnish).

Plant, R., Lesser, H. and Taylor-Gooby, P. (1980). *Political Philosophy and Social Welfare: Essays on the Normative Basis of Welfare Provision.* London, Routledge and Kegan Paul.

Polanyi, K. (1944). *The Great Transformation.* New York, Rinehard.

Porter, M. E. (1980). *Competitive Advantage.* New York, Free Press.

Praktikertjänst AB (1980). *A Swedish Service Company for Private Practitioners.* Stockholm, Pratktikerjänst AB.

Praktikertjänst AB (1987). *Årsredovisning 1986/1987.* Stockholm, Praktikertjänst AB.

Pressman, J. and Wildavsky, A. (1973). *Implementation.* Berkeley, University of California Press.

Raimondo, M. (1991). 'Total quality management and health care', University of Massachusetts/Amherst seminar paper.

Regeringens skrivelse (1984/5). *Den offentliga sektorns förnyelse.* Stockholm.

Robinson, R. (1988). *Increasing Efficiency in Clinical Services: a Case for the Internal Market?* London, Institute for Economic Studies.

Rosenthal, M. (1986). 'Beyond equity: Swedish health policy and the private sector', *Milbank Quarterly*, **64**, 592–621.

Rosenthal, M. (1990). 'Growth of private medicine in Sweden: the new diversity and the new challenge', paper delivered at Conference on Swedish Health Policy – a Comparative Perspective, Högberga, Lidingö, 22–24 August.

Rutten, F. F. H. (1986). 'Market strategies for publicly financed health care systems', *Health Policy*, **7**, 135–48.

Ryan, M. (1987). 'Remuneration of Soviet medical personnel', *British Medical Journal*, **294**, 1340–1.

Rydén, J. and Sjönell, G. (1989). 'Så avlastas akuten', *Svenska Dagbladet*, 25 July.

Saltman, R. B. (1985a). 'The capital-decision making process in regionalized health systems: some evidence from Sweden and Denmark', *Health Policy*, **4**, 279–89.

Saltman, R. B. (1985b). 'Power and cost containment in a Danish public hospital', *Journal of Health Politics, Policy and Law*, **9**, 563–94.

Saltman, R. B. (1986). 'Designing standardized clinical protocols: some organizational and behavioral issues', *International Journal of Health Planning and Management*, **1**, 129–41.

Saltman, R. B. (1987). 'Management control in a publicly planned health system: a case study from Finland', *Health Policy*, **8**, 283–98.

Saltman, R. B. (1988a). 'National planning for locally controlled health systems: the Finnish experience', *Journal of Health Politics, Policy and Law*, **13**, 27–51.

Saltman, R. B. (1988b). 'Health care in Sweden', in R. B. Saltman (ed.) *The International Handbook of Health Care Systems*. Westport, CT and London, Greenwood Press, pp. 285–93.

Saltman, R. B. (1990). 'Competition and reform in the Swedish health system', *Milbank Quarterly*, **68**, 597–618.

Saltman, R. B. and de Roo, A. (1989). 'Hospital policy in the Netherlands: the parameters of structural stalemate', *Journal of Health Politics, Policy and Law*, **14**, 773–95.

Saltman, R. B. and von Otter, C. (1987). 'Revitalizing public health care systems: a proposal for public competition in Sweden', *Health Policy*, **7**, 21–40.

Saltman, R. B. and von Otter, C. (1989a). 'Public competition vs. mixed markets: an analytic comparison', *Health Policy*, **11**, 43–55.

Saltman, R. B. and von Otter, C. (1989b). 'Voice, choice, and the question of civil democracy in the Swedish welfare state', *Economic and Industrial Democracy*, **10**, 195–209.

Saltman, R. B. and von Otter, C. (1990). 'Implementing public competition in Swedish county councils: a case study', *International Journal of Health Planning and Management*, **5**, 105–16.

Saltman, R. B., Harrison, S. and von Otter, C. (1991). 'Competition and public funds', *Hospital Management International*, annual edition, pp. 105–8.

Sapinski, W. (1988). *New Possibility to Choose a Doctor in Poland*. Łódź, Department of Social Medicine, Medical Academy.

Sapolsky, H. M. (1987). 'Prospective payment in perspective', *Journal of Health Politics, Policy and Law*, **11**, 633–46.

SCB (1988). *Hälsan i Sverige: Hälsostatistisk årsbok 1987/88*. Stockholm, Statistiska Centralbyrån.

Schieber, G. and Poullier, J. P. (1989). 'International health care expenditure trends: 1987', *Health Affairs*, **8**, 169–77.

Schieber, G. and Poullier, J.-P. (1991). 'International health spending: issues and trends', *Health Affairs*, **10**, 106–16.

Schildt, A. (1988). 'In Sweden, equality is tinged with inefficiency', *Washington Post*, 16 August.

Schlesinger, M., Marmor, T. R. and Smithy, R. (1987). 'Non-profit and for-profit medical care: shifting the roles and implications of health policy', *Journal of Health Politics, Policy and Law*, **12**, 427–57.

Schumpeter, J. A. (1934). *The Theory of Economic Development: an Inquiry into Profits, Capital, Credit, Interest, and the Business Cycle*. Harvard Economic Studies, Vol. 46. Cambridge, MA, Harvard University Press. First published as *Theorie der wirtschaftlichen Entwicklung* (1912).

Scrivens, E. (1988). 'Consumers, accountability, and quality of service', in R. Maxwell (ed.) *Reshaping the National Health Service*. London: Policy Journals, pp. 170–87.

Serner, U. (1980). 'Swedish health legislation: milestones in reorganization since 1945', in A. J. Heidenheimer and N. J. Elvander (eds) *The Shaping of the Swedish Health Care System*. New York: St Martin's, pp. 99–116.

SIAR (1990). *Människor i Samspel*. Lund, SIAR (mimeo).

Sitkery, I. (1989). 'Problems and perspectives of the Hungarian health system', paper delivered at the Annual Conference of the European Healthcare Management Association, Helsinki, Finland.

Socialstyrelsen (1988). *Köer i sjukvården: Sammanfattande redovisning och uppföljning effektiverna av statsbidraget*. Stockholm, Socialstyrelsen.

SOU (1985). *Aktivt folkstyre i kommuner och landsting. Betänkande från 1983 års demokratiberedning*. Stockholm, SOU.

Stenberg, G. and Åhgren, B. (1987). *Primärvårdens effektivitet*. Göteborg, AB Spri-konsult.

Stoddart, G. L. and Seldon, J. R. (1983). 'Publicly financed competition in Canadian health care delivery: a viable alternative to increased regulation?', in J. A. Boan (ed.) *Proceedings of the Second Canadian Conference on Health Economics; Health Insurance: a Silver Anniversary Appraisal*. Regina, Saskatchewan, University of Regina.

Strong, P. and Robinson, J. (1990). *The NHS under New Management*. Milton Keynes and Philadelphia, Open University Press.

Stryjan, Y. (1989). *Impossible Organizations: On Self Management and Organizational Reproduction*. Westport, CT, Greenwood Press.

Svensson, L. (1986). *Grupper och kollektiv. En undersökning av hemtjänstens organisation i två kommuner*. Stockholm, Arbetslivscentrum.

Tengvald, K. (1981). *Arbetsning och ledning i vårdlag*. Stockholm, Arbetslivscentrum.

Västsvenska Planeringsnämnden (1984). *Regionsjukvårdsavtal med därtill knutna avtal för västra sjukvårdsregionen*. Göteborg, Västsvenska Planeringsnämnden.

Vohlonen, I. and Pekurinen, M. (1990). *Variation in Hospital Productivity: Effects of Planning, Administration and Monitoring*. Helsinki, National Board of Health.

Vohlonen, I., Pekurinen, M. and Saltman, R. B. (1989). 'Reorganizing primary medical care in Finland: the personal doctor program', *Health Policy*, **13**, 65–79.

von Otter, C. (ed.) (1983). *Worker Participation in the Public Sector*. Stockholm, Almquist and Wiksell International.

von Otter, C. (1986a). *Den effektiva förvaltningen*. Stockholm, TCO.

von Otter, C. (1986b). *Kan man rationalisera folkhemmet?* Eskiltuna, Tuna Tryck.

von Otter, C. (1988). 'Responsiveness in public service organizations, the case for "public competition", and "participative management"', paper delivered at the OECD Workshop on Urban Services and Consumer Needs, Amsterdam, April 22–25. Stockholm, Swedish Centre for Working Life.

von Otter, C. (1991). 'The application of market principles to health care', in Proceedings of EHMA Conference on Paradoxes of Competition, Nuffield Institute, University of Leeds.

von Otter, C. and Saltman, R. B. (1988). 'Vitalisering av den offentliga sjukvården – Ett förslag till institutionell konkurrens', *Läkartidningen*, **85**, 2816–23.

von Otter, C. and Saltman, R. B. (1991). 'Towards a Swedish health policy for the 1990s: planned markets and public firms', *Social Science and Medicine*, **32**, 473–81.

von Otter, C., Saltman, R. B. and Joelsson, L. (1989). 'Valmöjligheter, konkurrens, entreprenader, mm, inom landstingens sjukvård – enkätresultat', Working paper, Swedish Centre for Working Life, Stockholm.

Waerness, K. (1984). 'The rationality of caring', *Economic and Industrial Democracy*, **5**, 185–211.

Warner, M. (1989). *The NHS White Paper: Born of Europe 1992*. Cardiff (mimeo).

Weale, A. (1985). 'Why are we waiting? The problem of unresponsiveness in the public social services', in R. Klein and M. Higgins (eds) *The Future of Welfare*. Oxford, Basil Blackwell, pp. 150–65.

Weber, M. (1947). *The Theory of Social and Economic Organization*, trans. and ed. A. M. Henderson and T. Parsons. New York, Free Press.

Whiteis, D. and Salmon, J. W. (1987). 'The proprietization of health care and the underdevelopment of the public sector', *International Journal of Health Services*, **17**, 47–64.

WHO (1984). *Regional Targets in Support of the Regional Strategy for Health for All*. Copenhagen, World Health Organization.

WHO (1989). *The Leningrad Experiment in Health Care Management 1988*. Copenhagen, World Health Organization.

WHO (1990). *Leningrad Revisited: Report of a Second Visit to the USSR*. Copenhagen, World Health Organization.

Wickings, I. and Child, T. (1988). 'Managing the estate', in R. Maxwell (ed.) *Reshaping the National Health Service*. London, Policy Journals, pp. 114–25.

Williamson, O. E. (1975). *Markets and Hierarchies: Analysis and Antitrust Implications*. New York, Free Press.

Williamson, O. E. (1985). *The Economic Institutions of Capitalism*. New York, Free Press.

Williamson, O. E. (1986). *Economic Organization: Firms, Markets and Policy Control*. Brighton, Wheatsheaf.

Williamson, O. E. and Ouchi, W. C. (1981). 'The markets and hierarchies and visible hand perspectives', in A. A. van de Ven and W. F. Joyce (eds) *Perspectives in Organizational Design*. New York, Wiley, pp. 347–70.

Wistow, G. (1988). 'Off-loading responsibilities for care', in R. Maxwell (ed.) *Reshaping the National Health Service*. London, Policy Journals, pp. 153–69.

Wolf, C. Jr (1988). *Markets or Governments: Choosing between Imperfect Alternatives*. Cambridge, MA, MIT Press.

Wolin, S. (1960). *Politics and Vision: Continuity and Innovation in Western Political Thought*. Boston: Little Brown Co.

Wortman, P., Vinokur, M. A. and Sechrest, L. (1988). 'Do consensus conferences work? A process evaluation of the NIH consensus development program', *Journal of Health Politics, Policy and Law*, **13**, 469–98.

Yates, J. (1987). *Why Are We Waiting? An Analysis of Hospital Waiting Lists*. Oxford, Oxford University Press.

Young, D. W. and Saltman, R. B. (1985). *The Hospital Power Equilibrium: Physician Behavior and Cost Control*. Baltimore, MD, Johns Hopkins University Press.

Zuidema, G. (1980). 'The problem of cost containment in teaching hospitals: the Johns Hopkins experience', *Surgery*, **87**, 41–4.

INDEX